Keep Calm And Color Dicks

A FUNNY DICK COLORING BOOK FOR ADULTS

ROCCO VIDAL

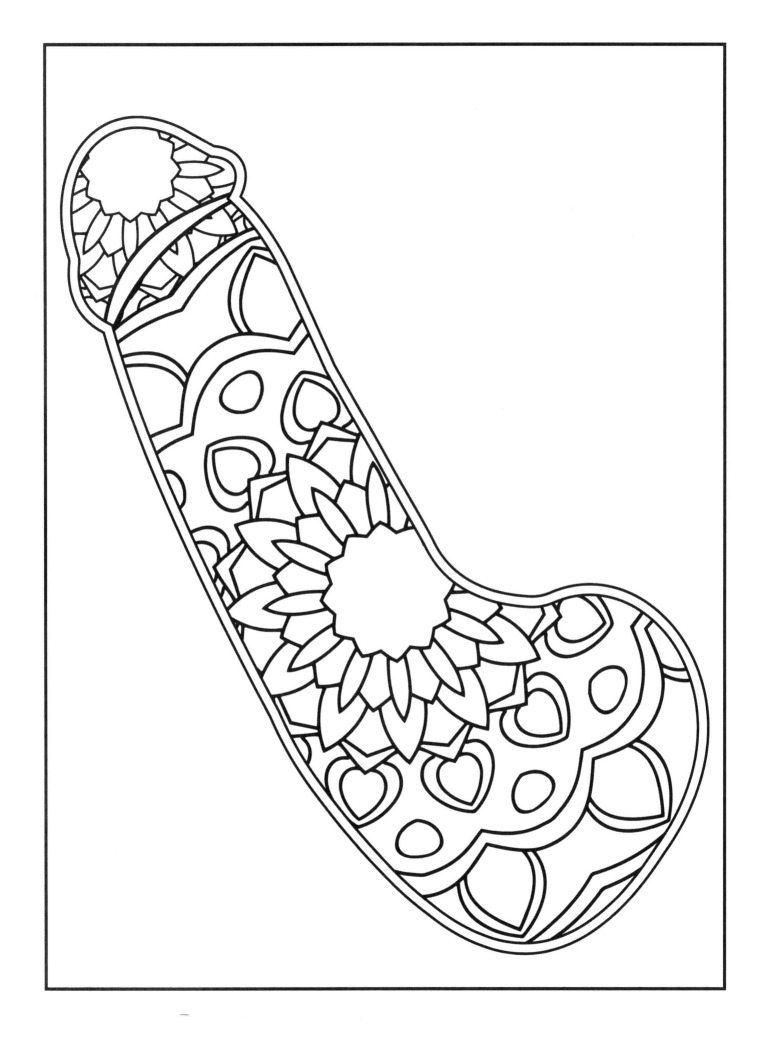

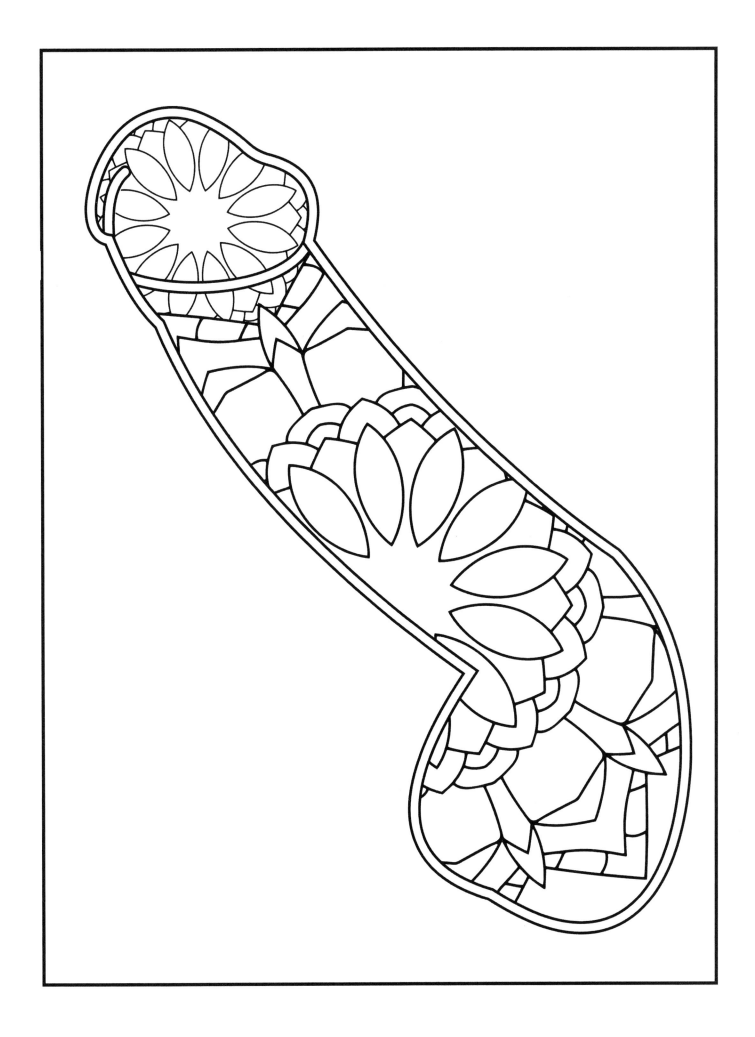

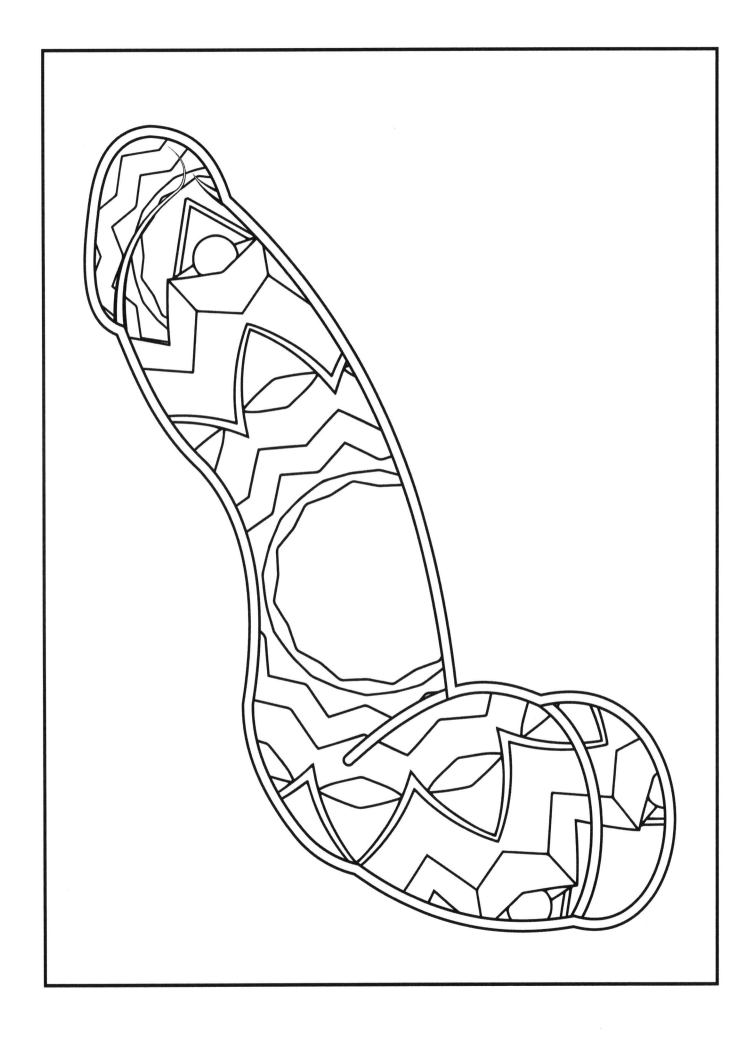

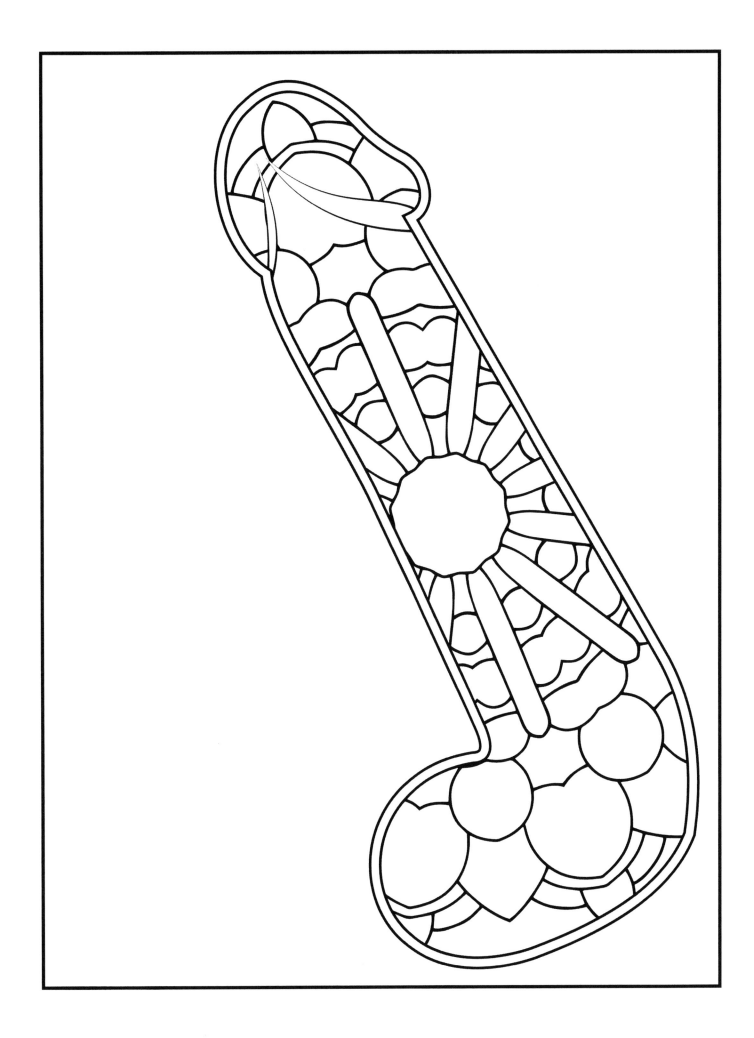

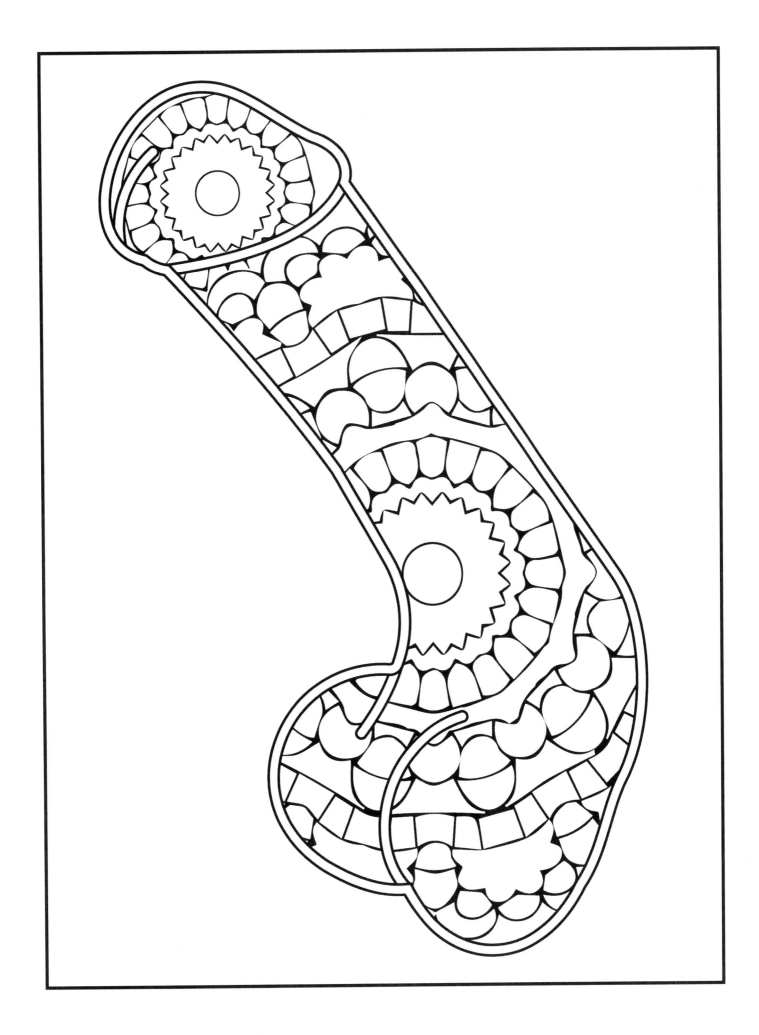

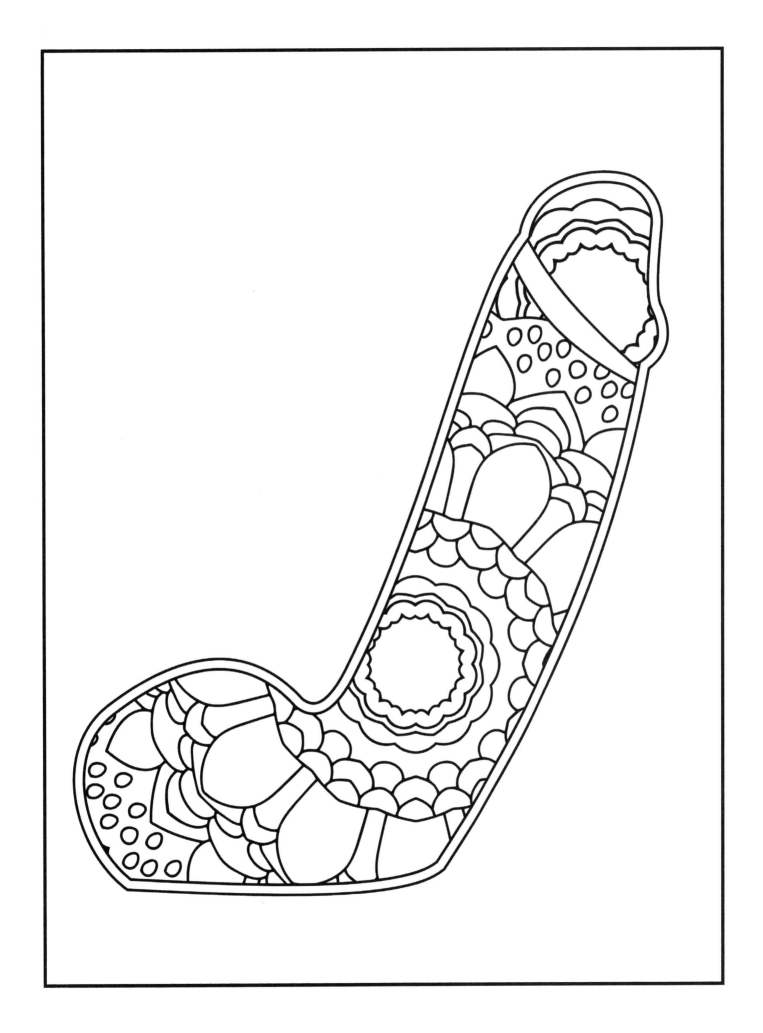

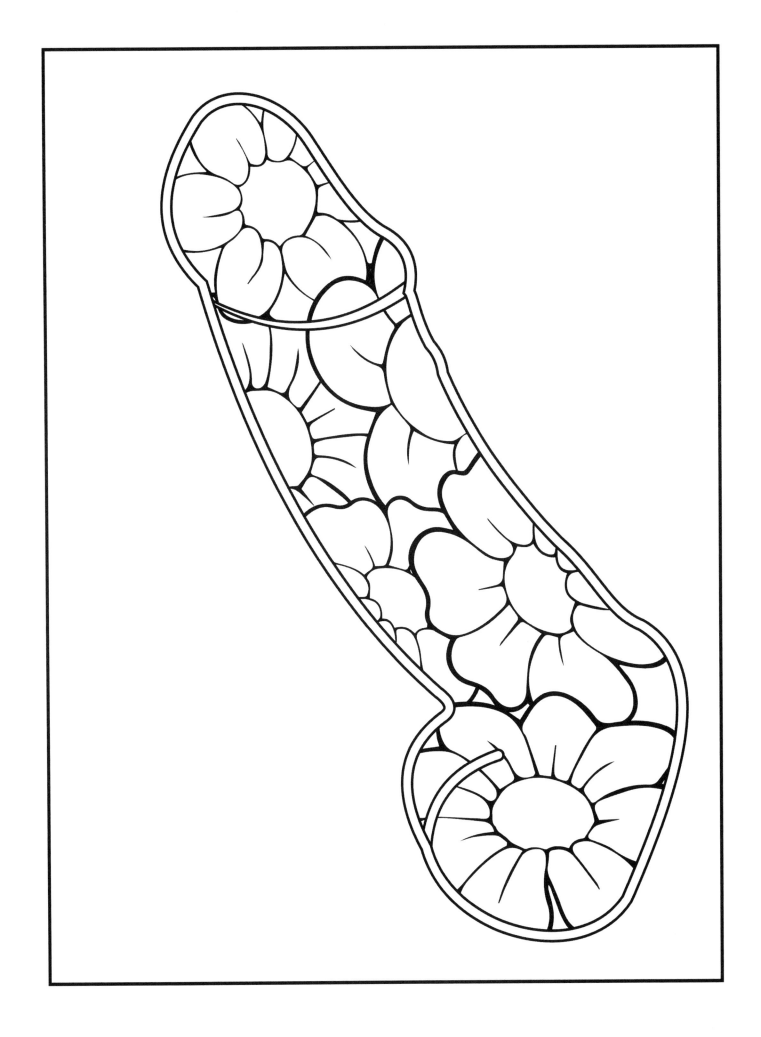

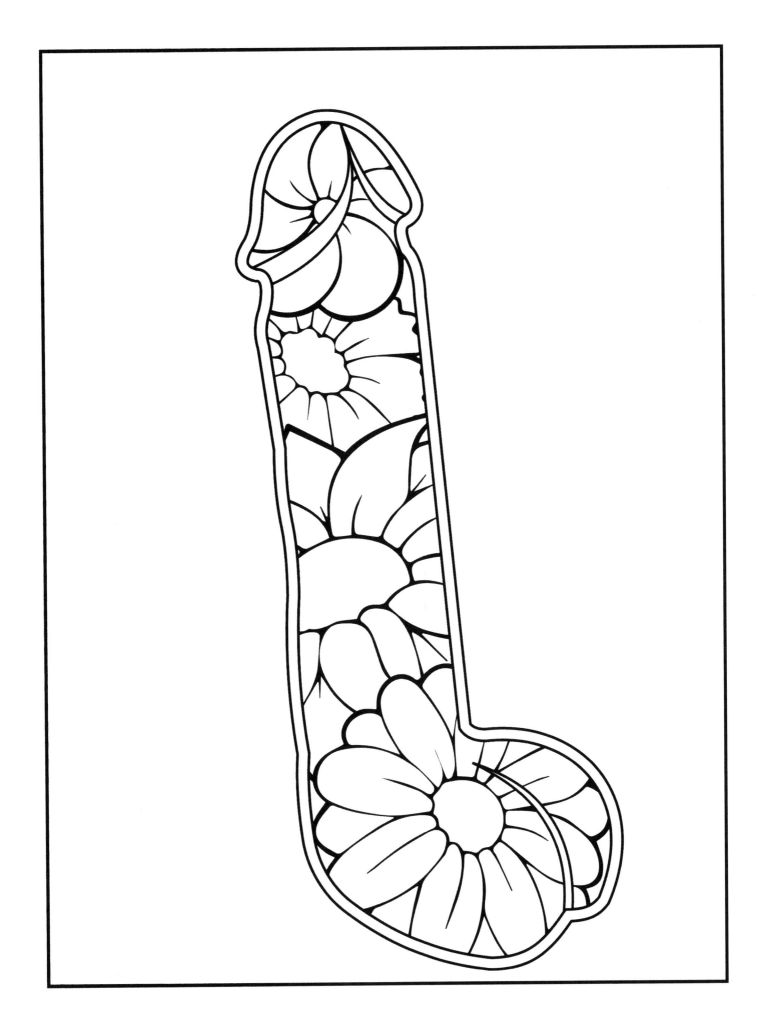

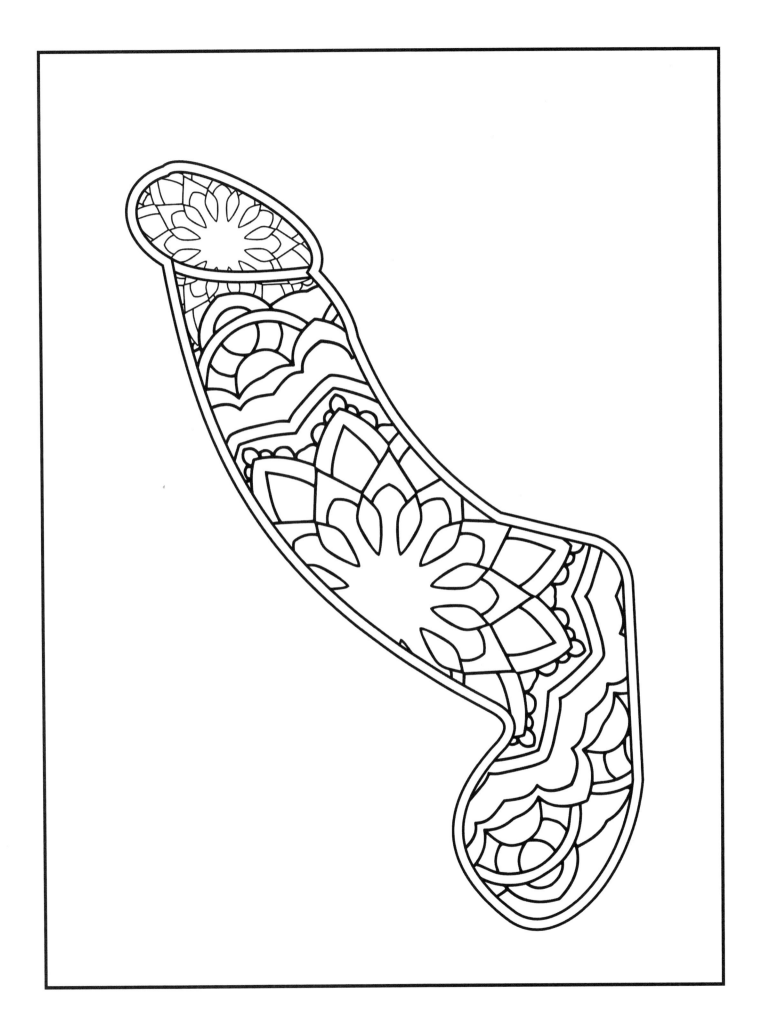

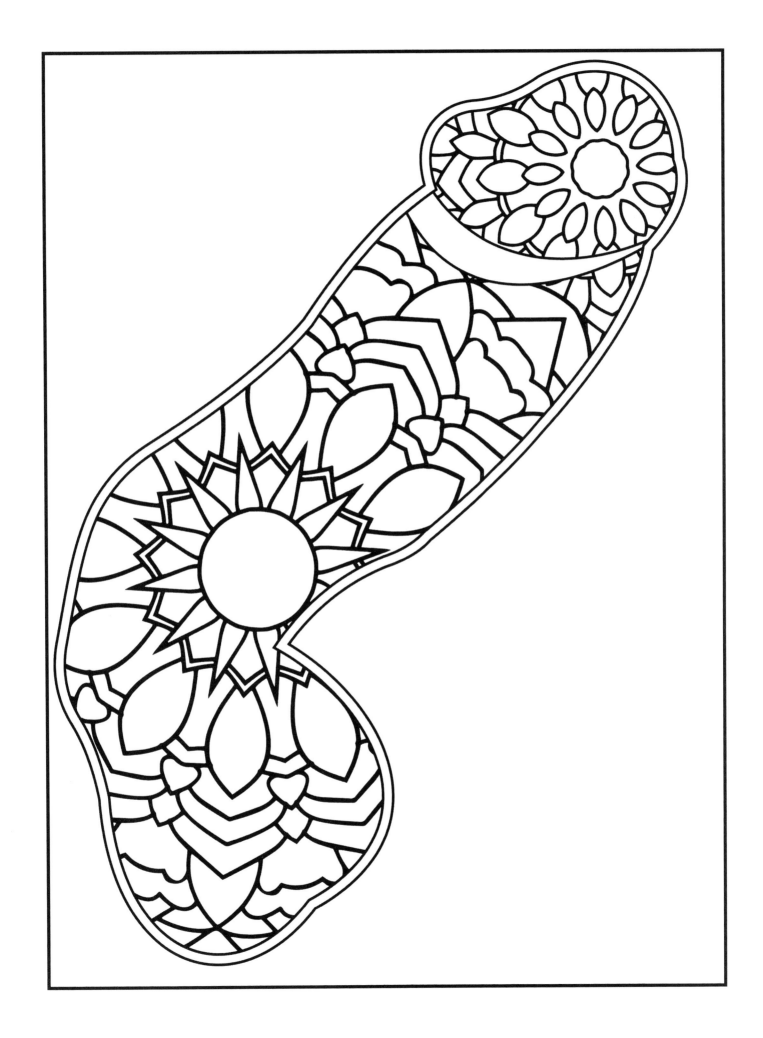

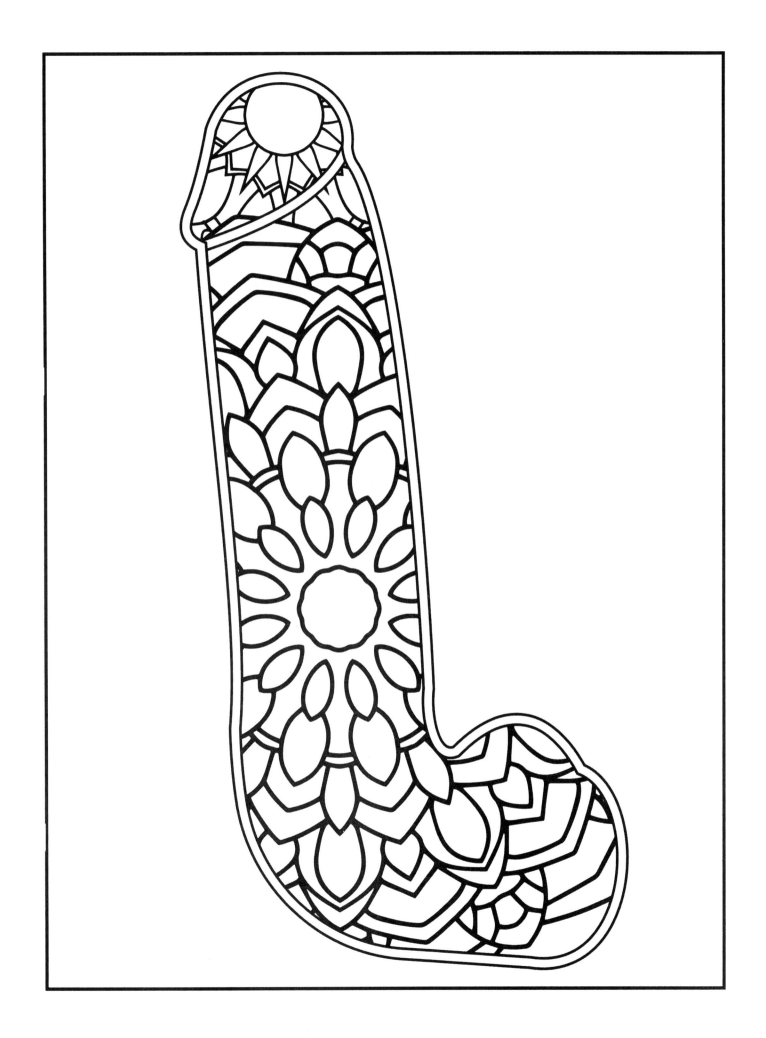

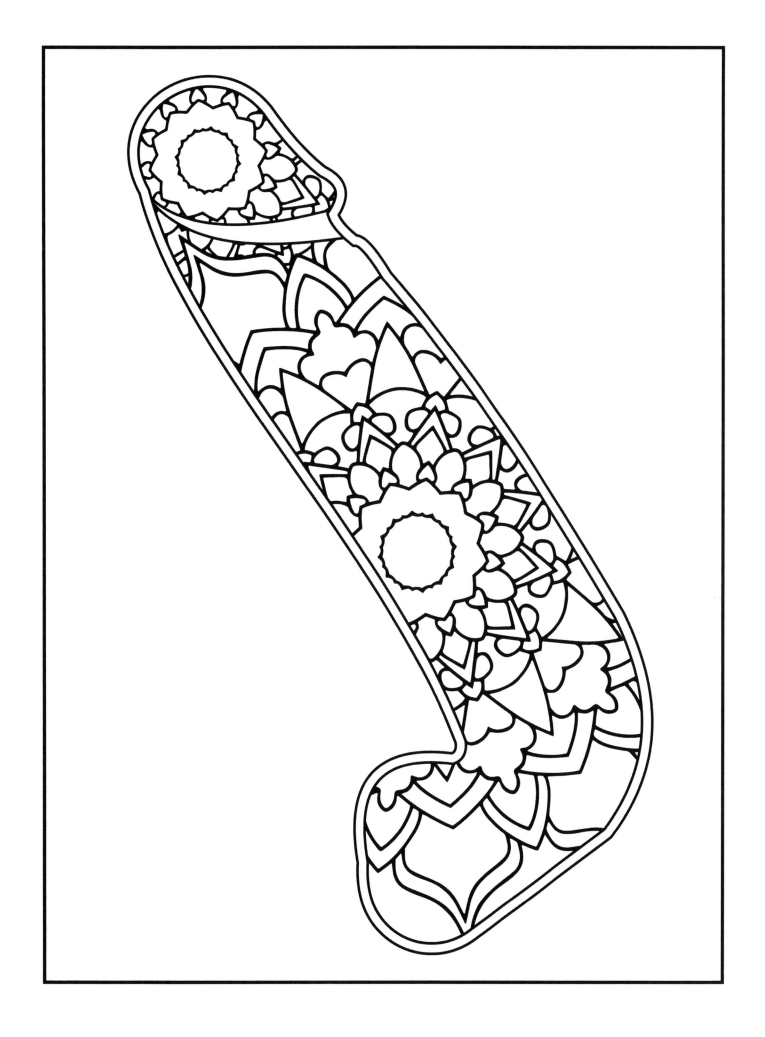

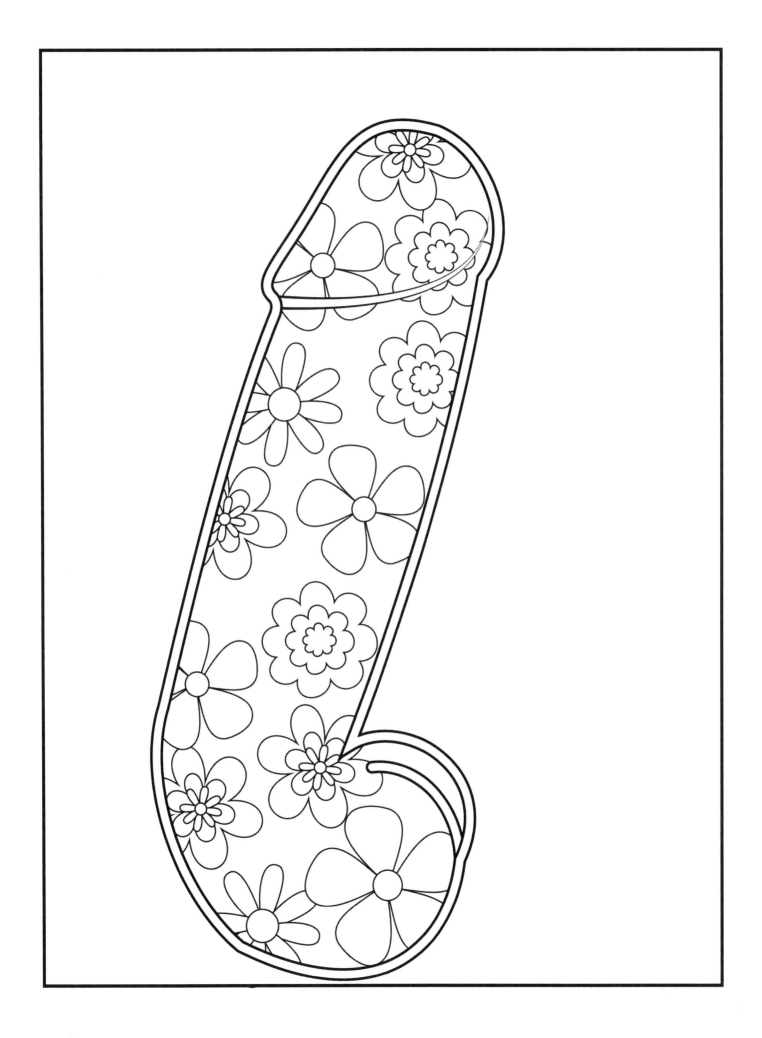

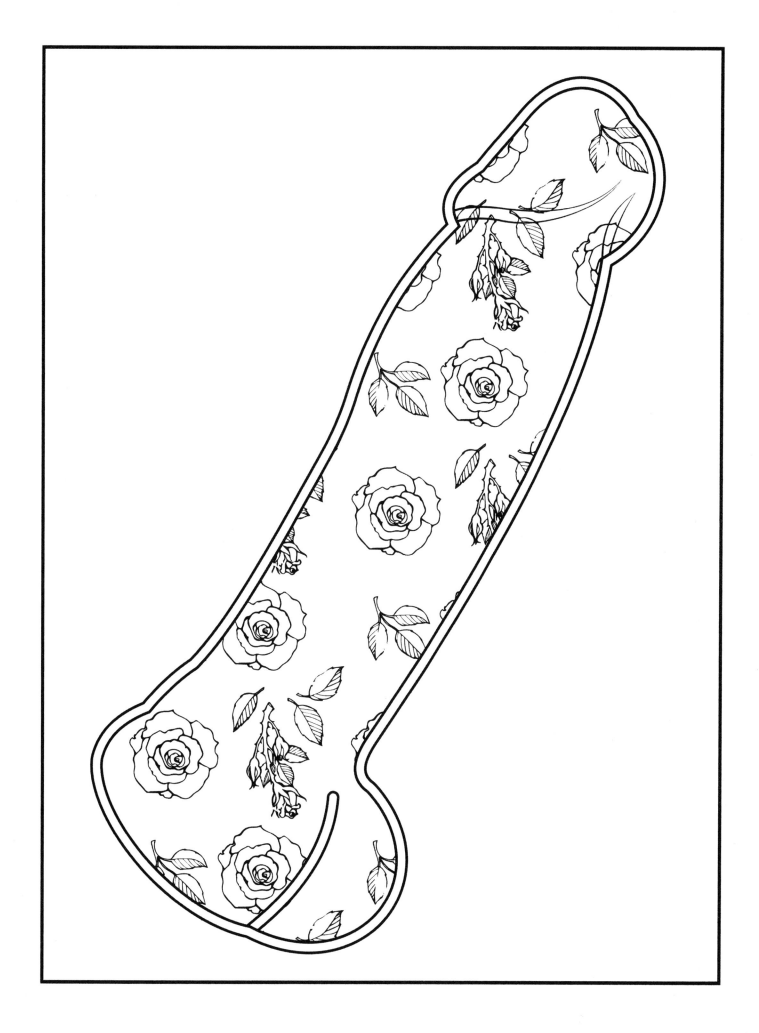

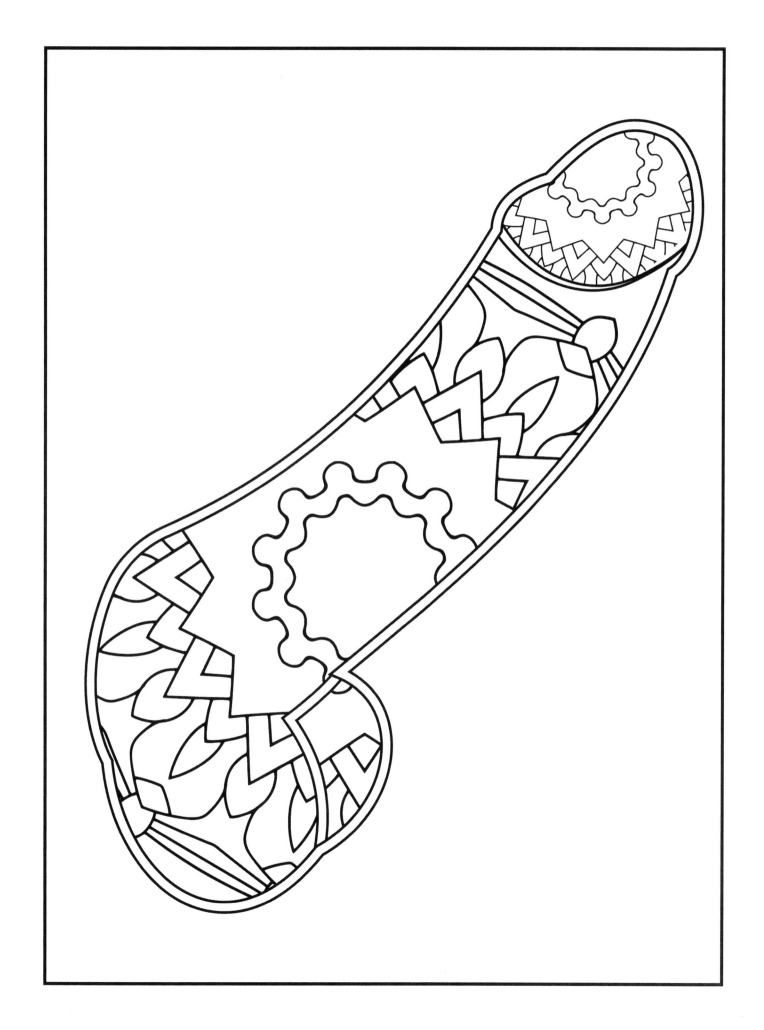

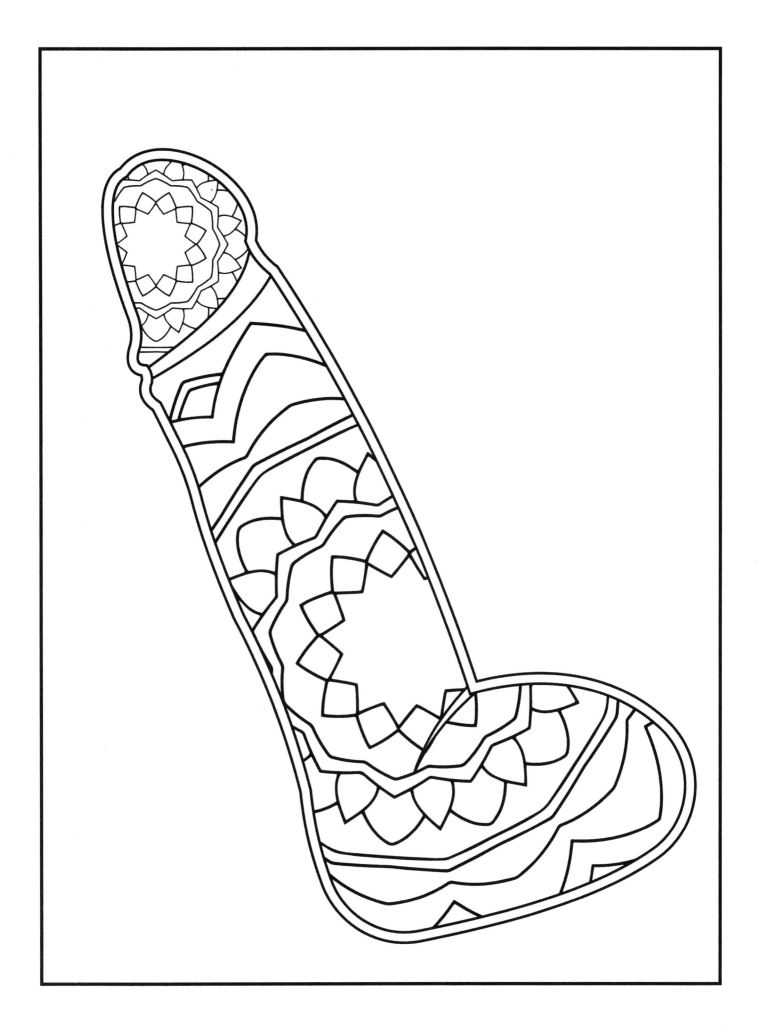

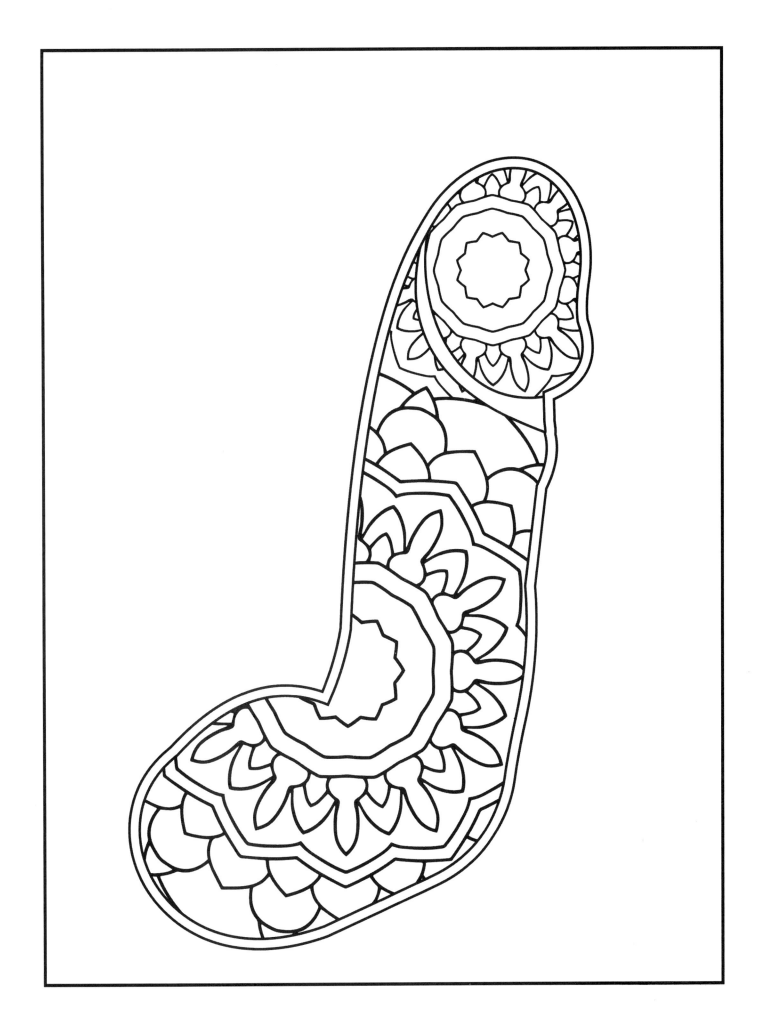

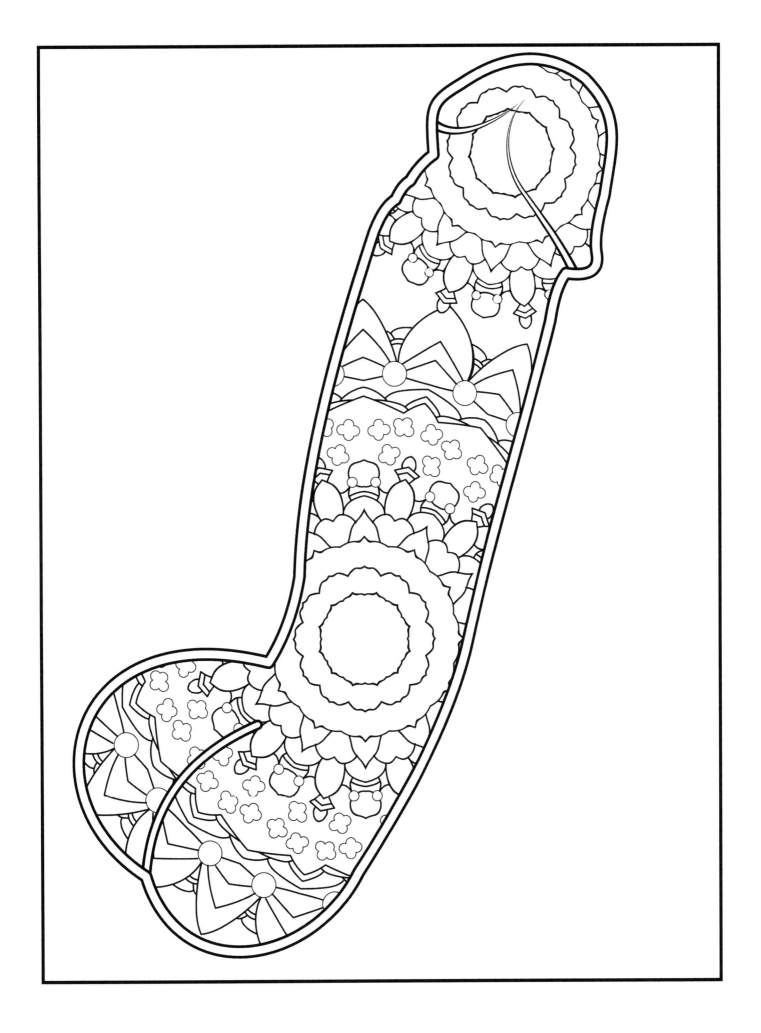

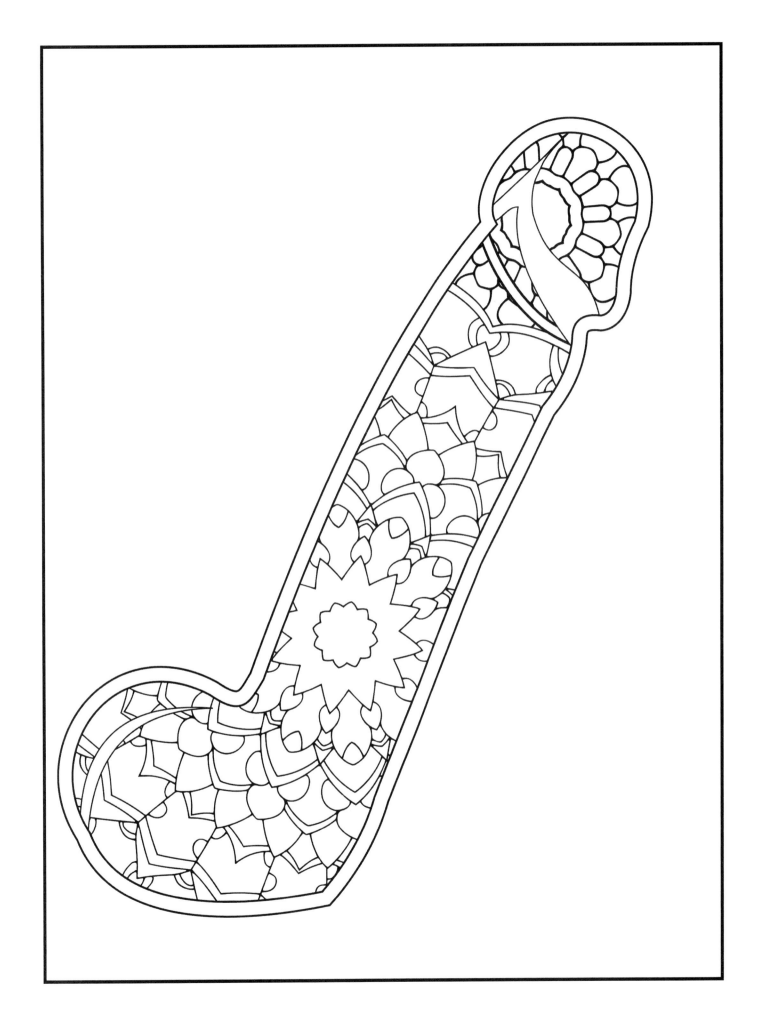

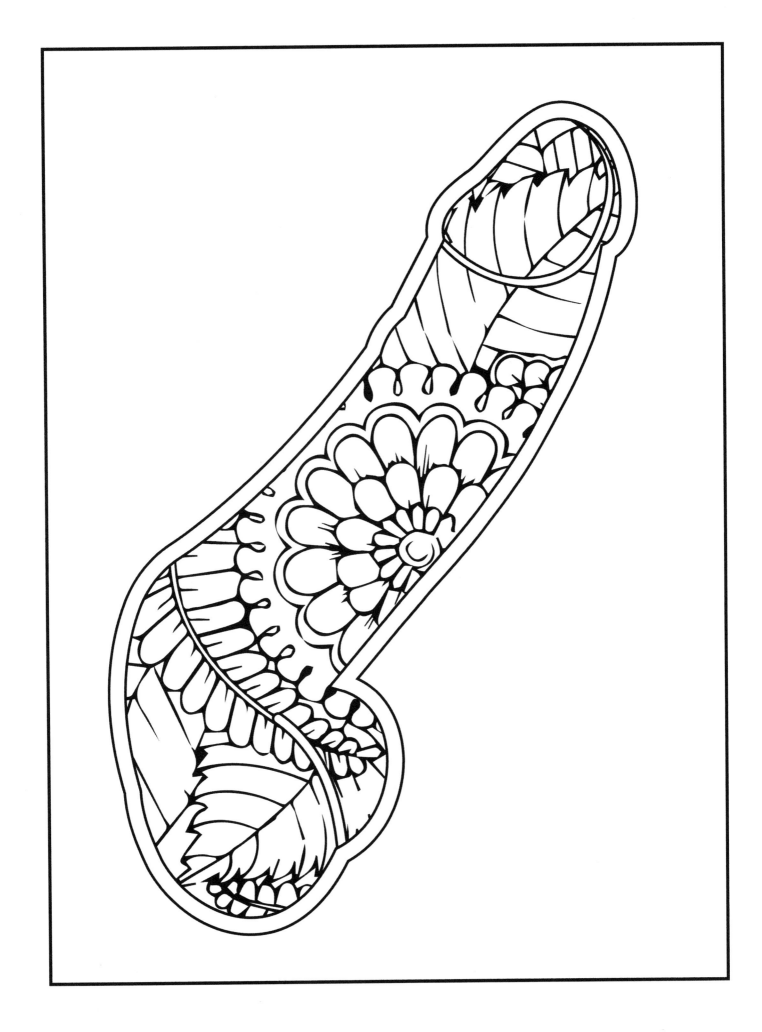

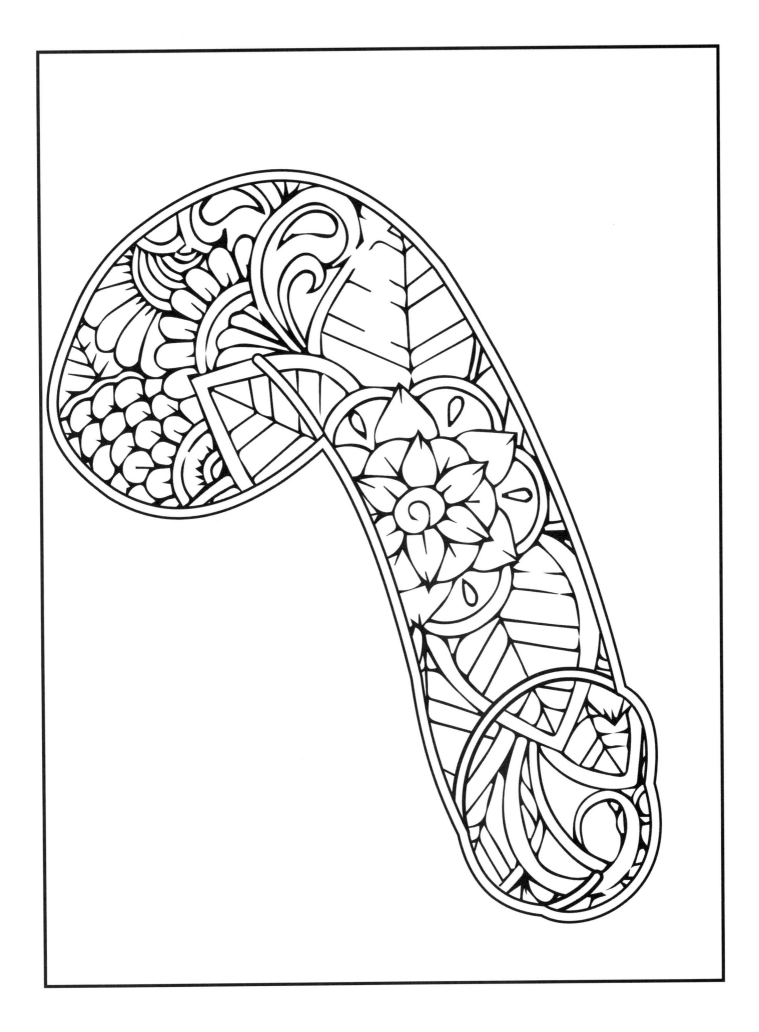

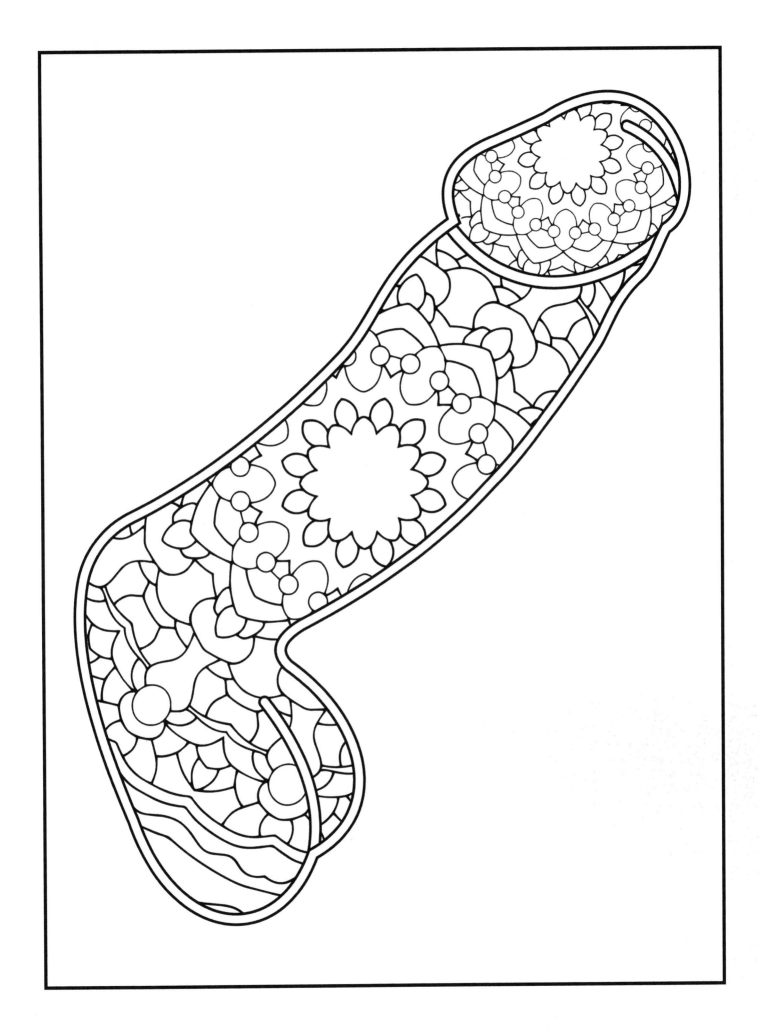

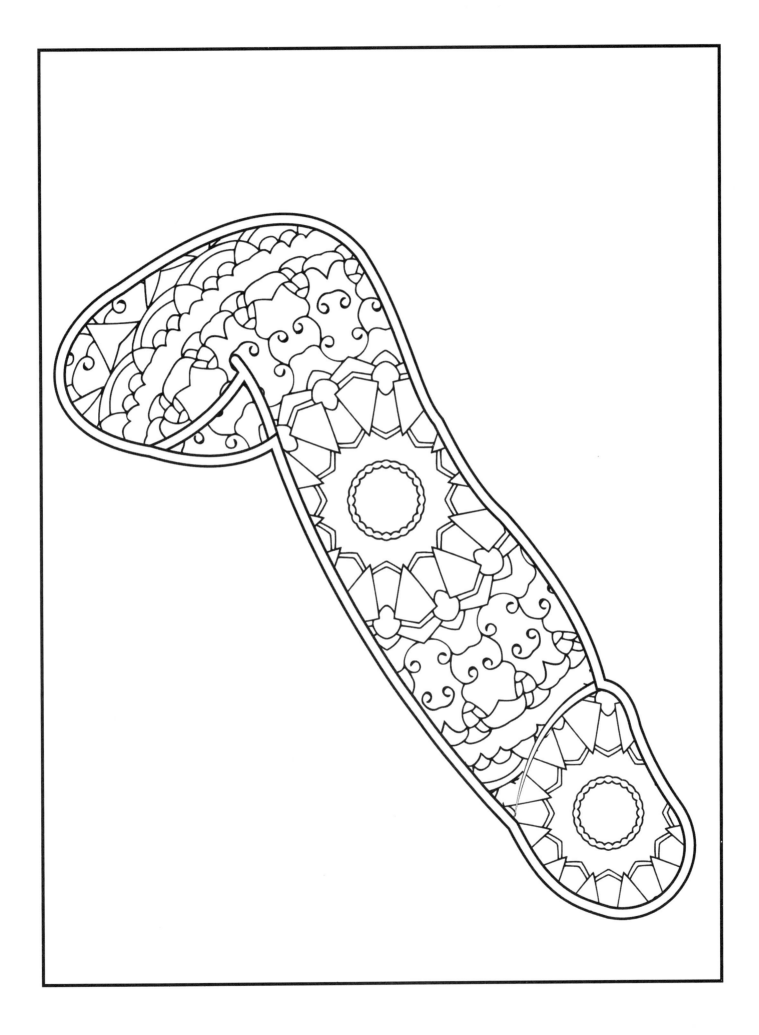

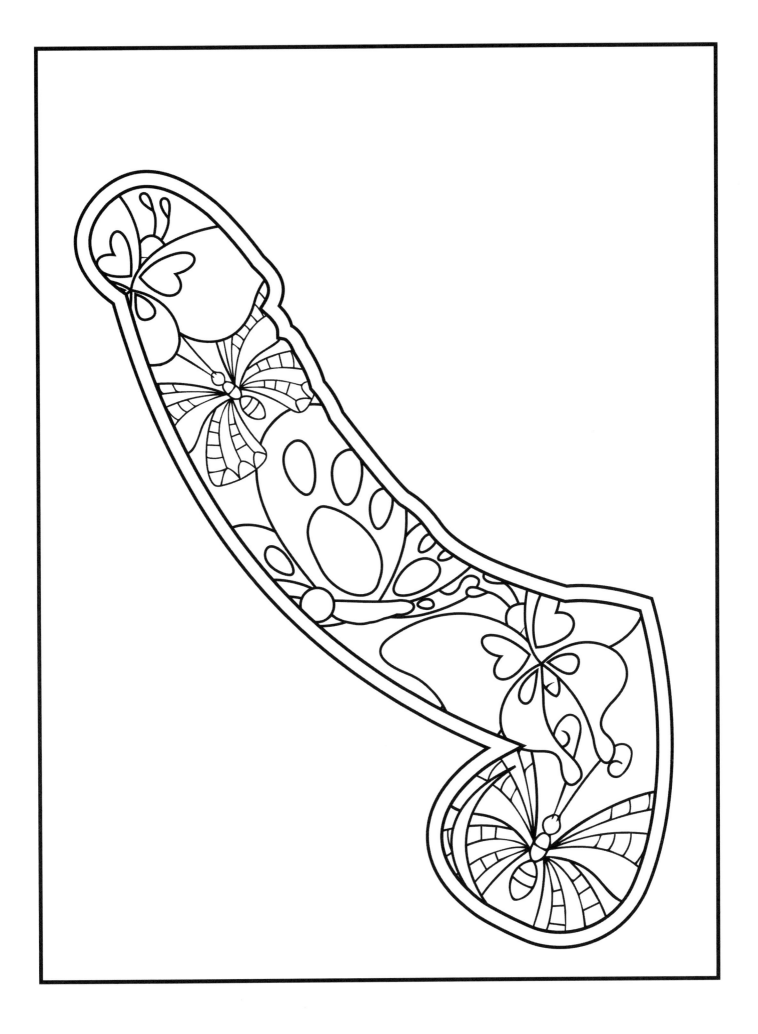

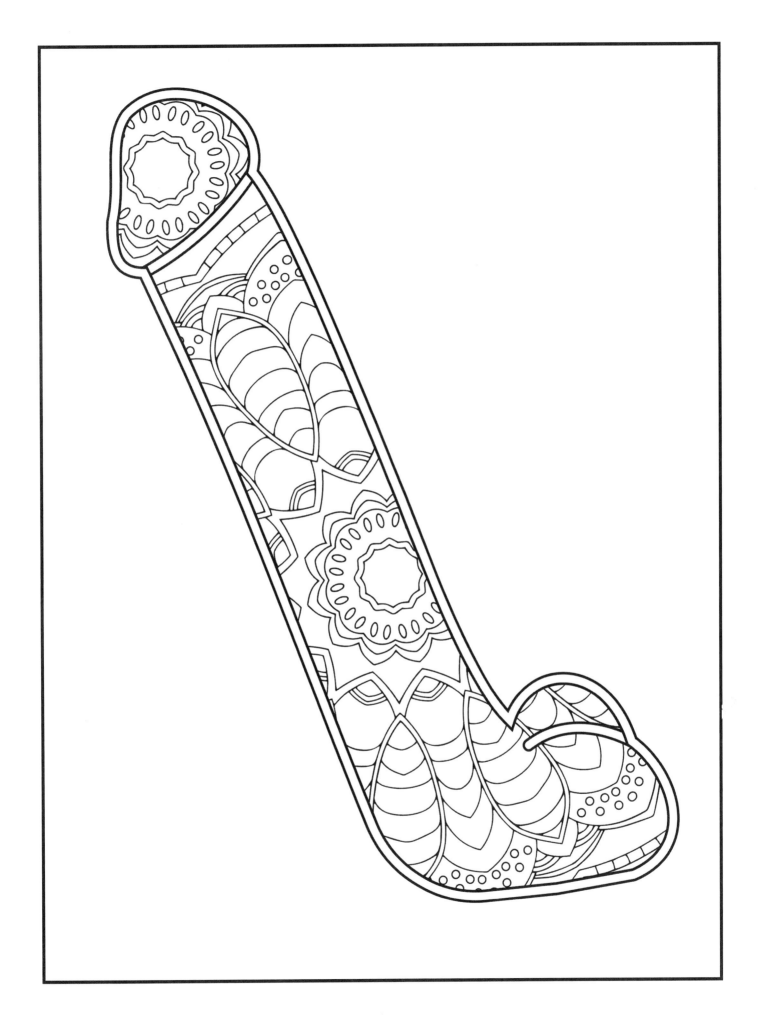

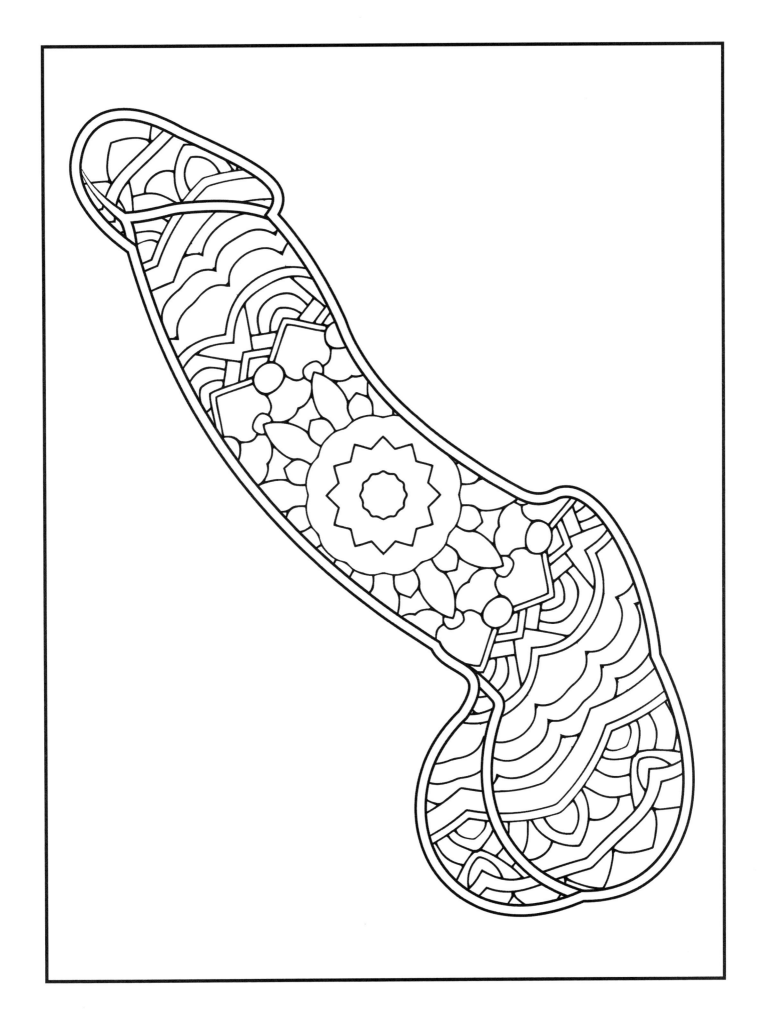

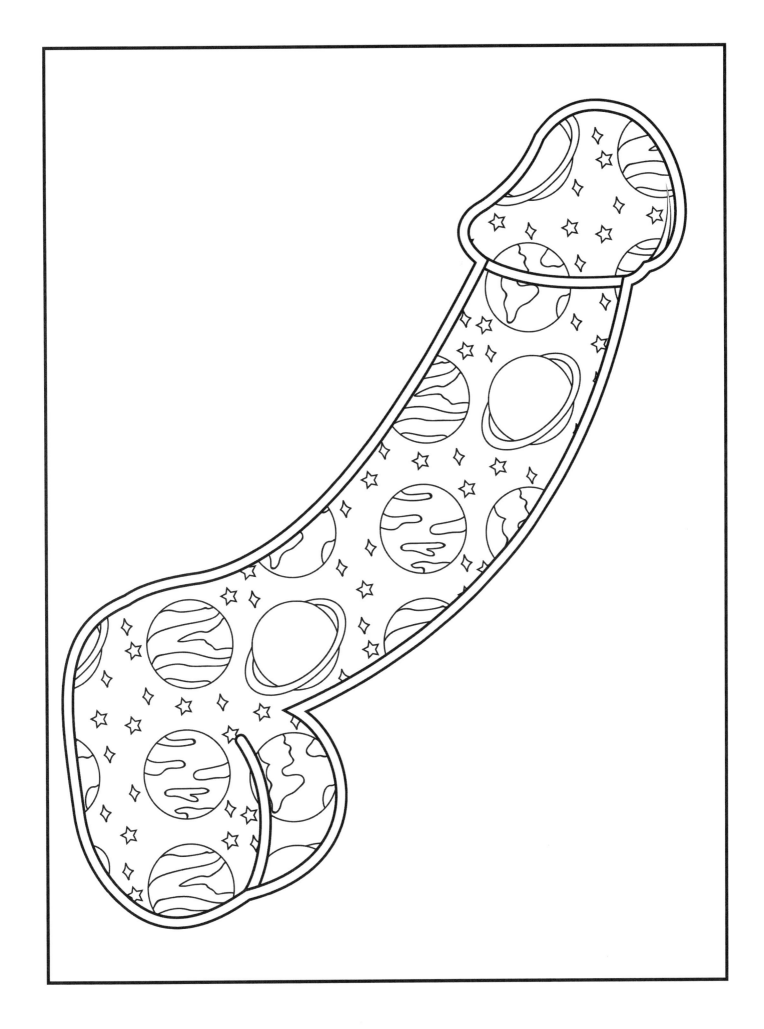

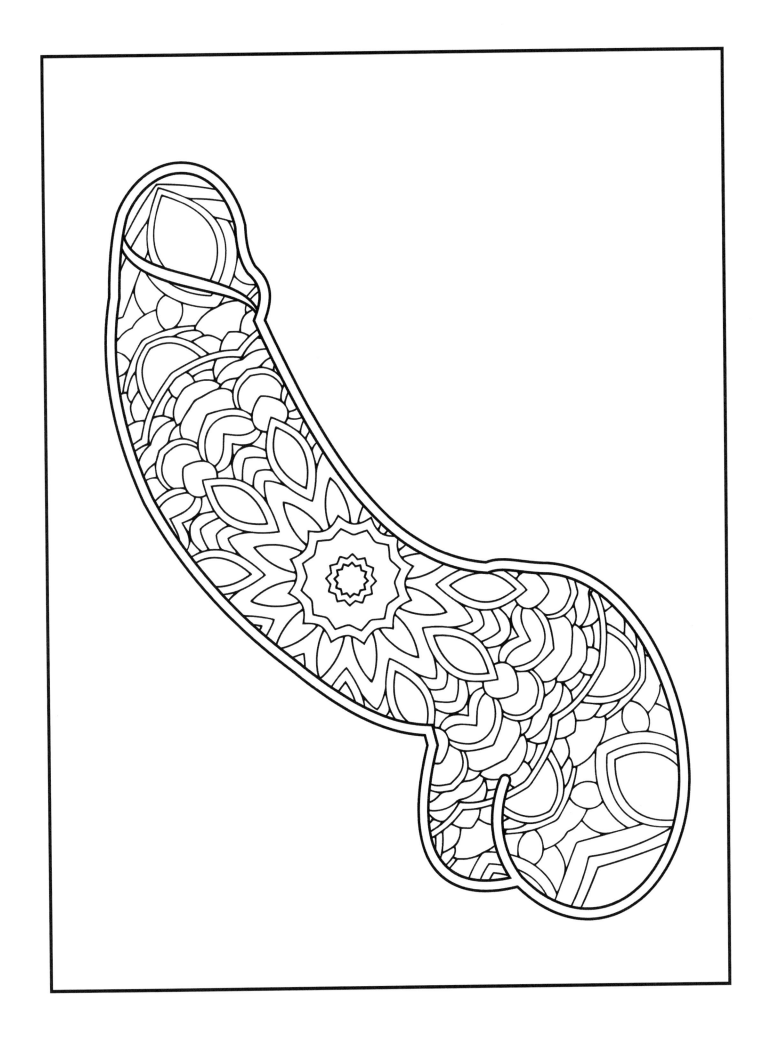

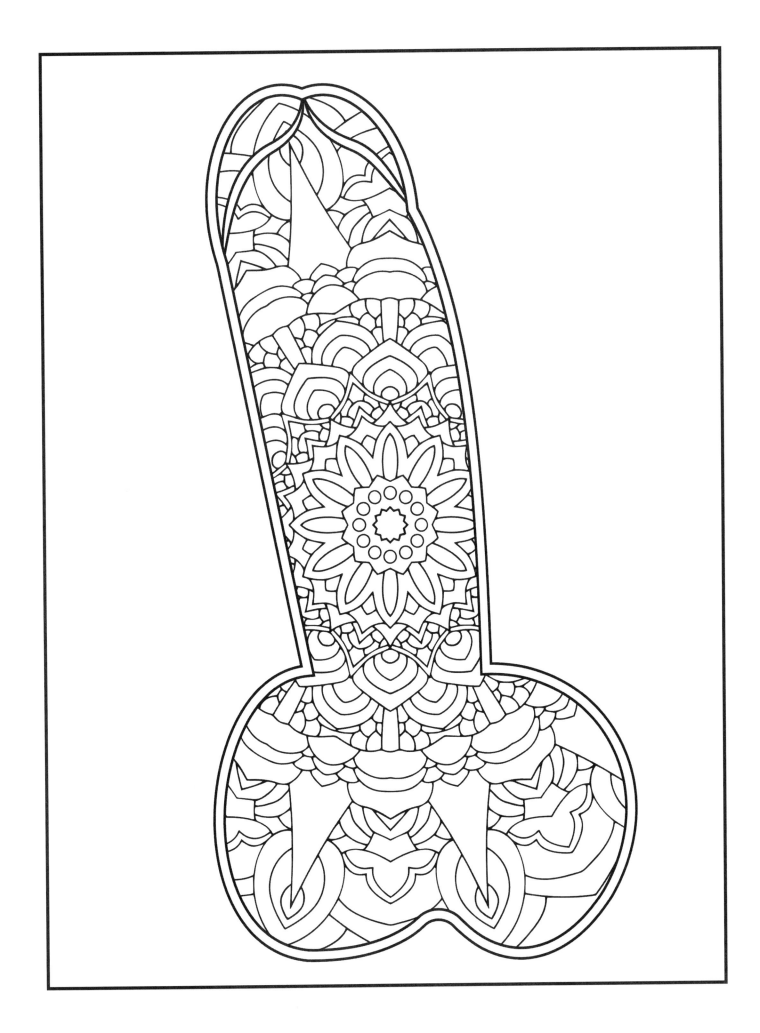

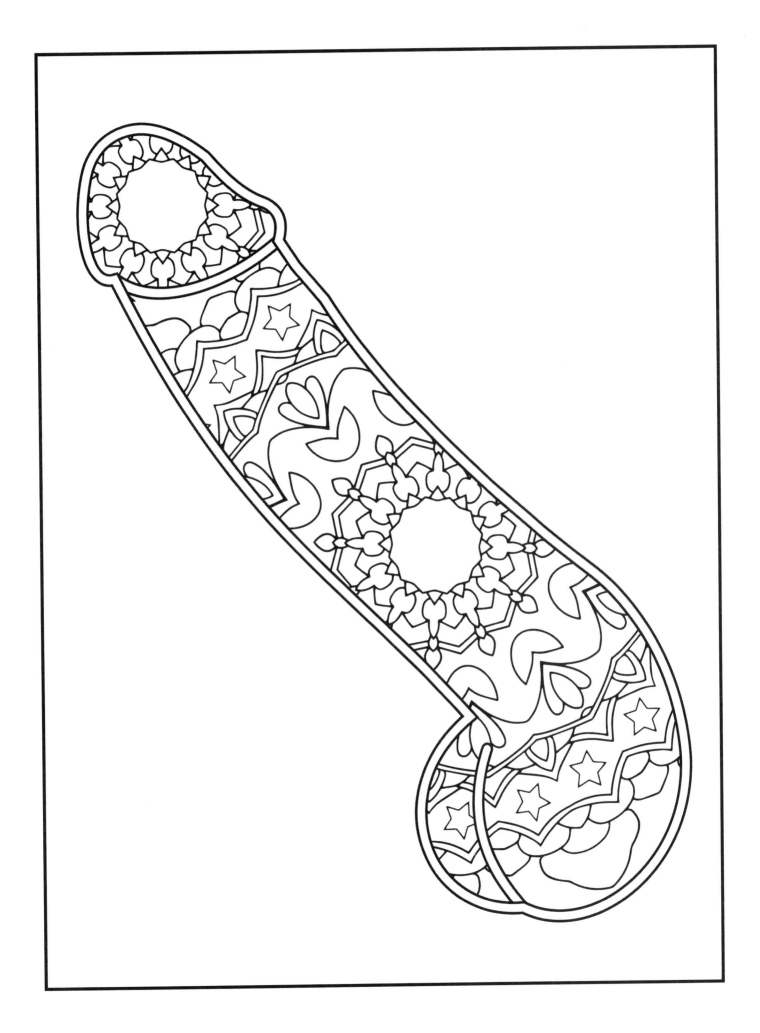

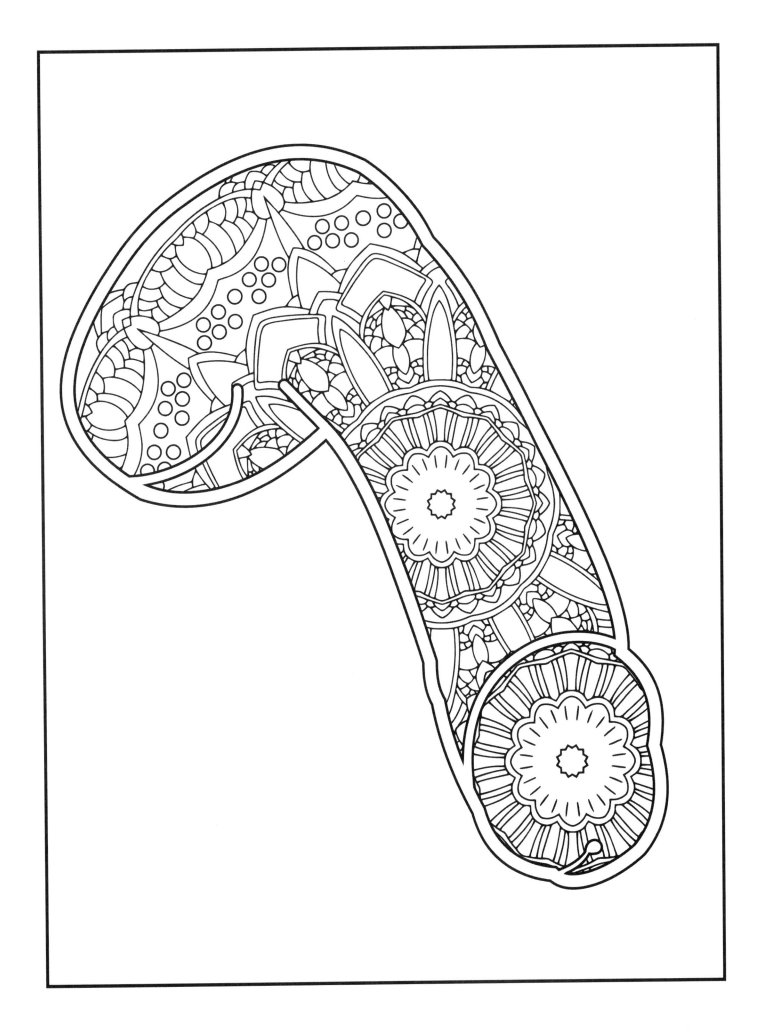

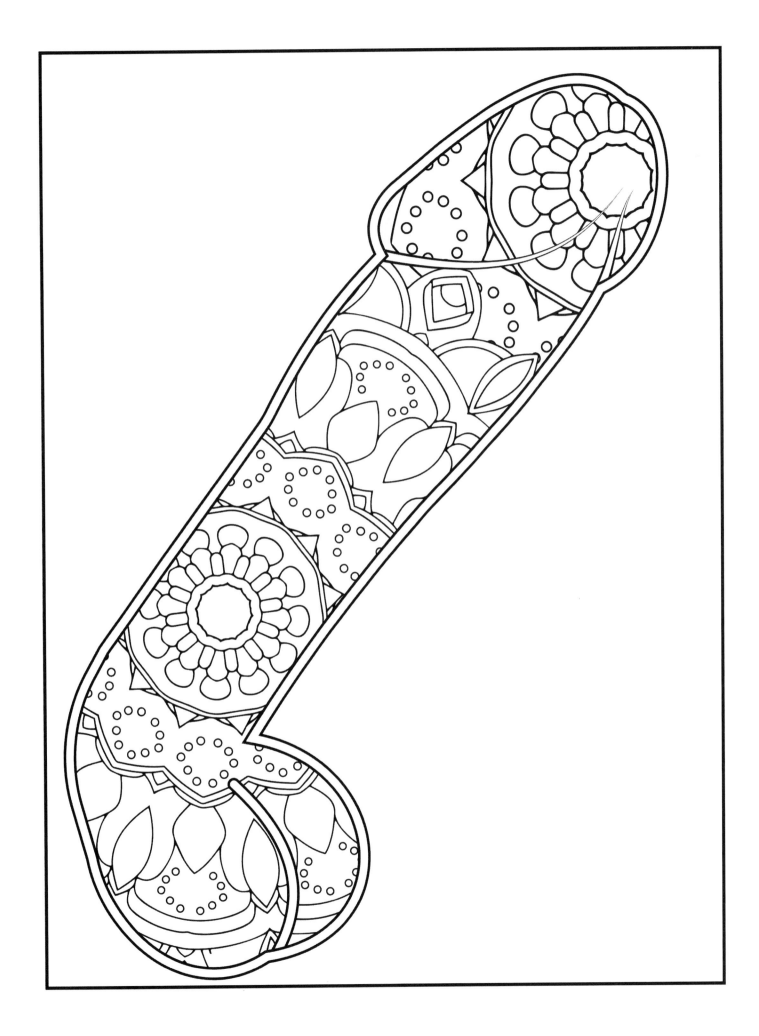

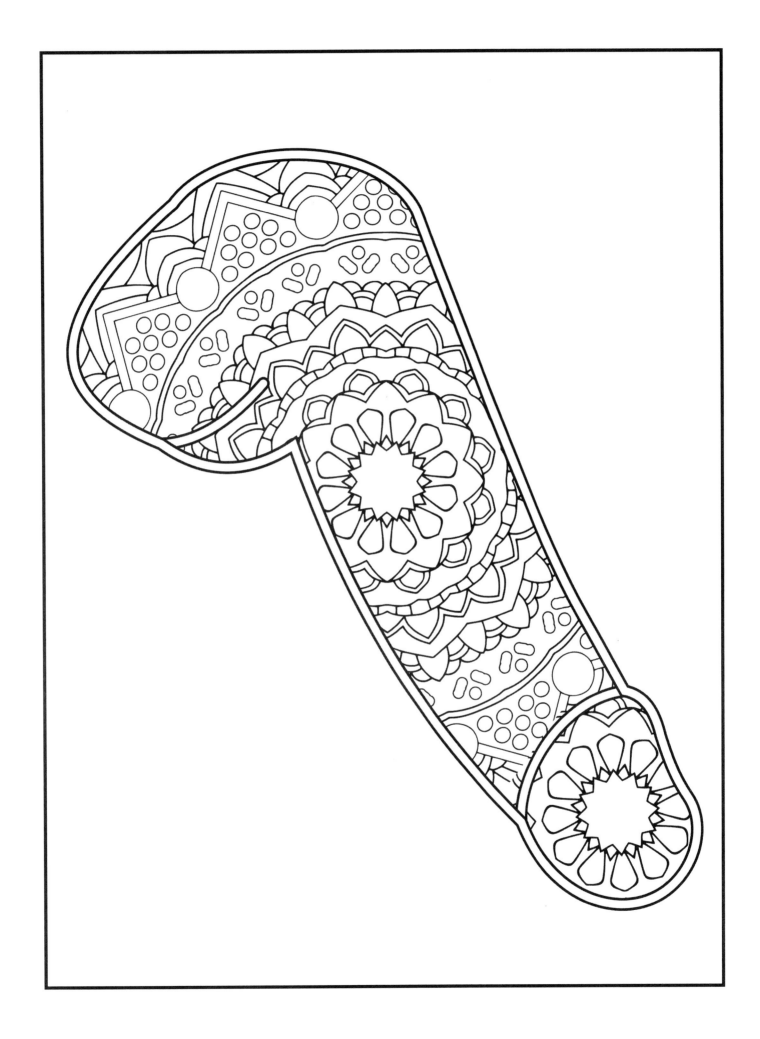

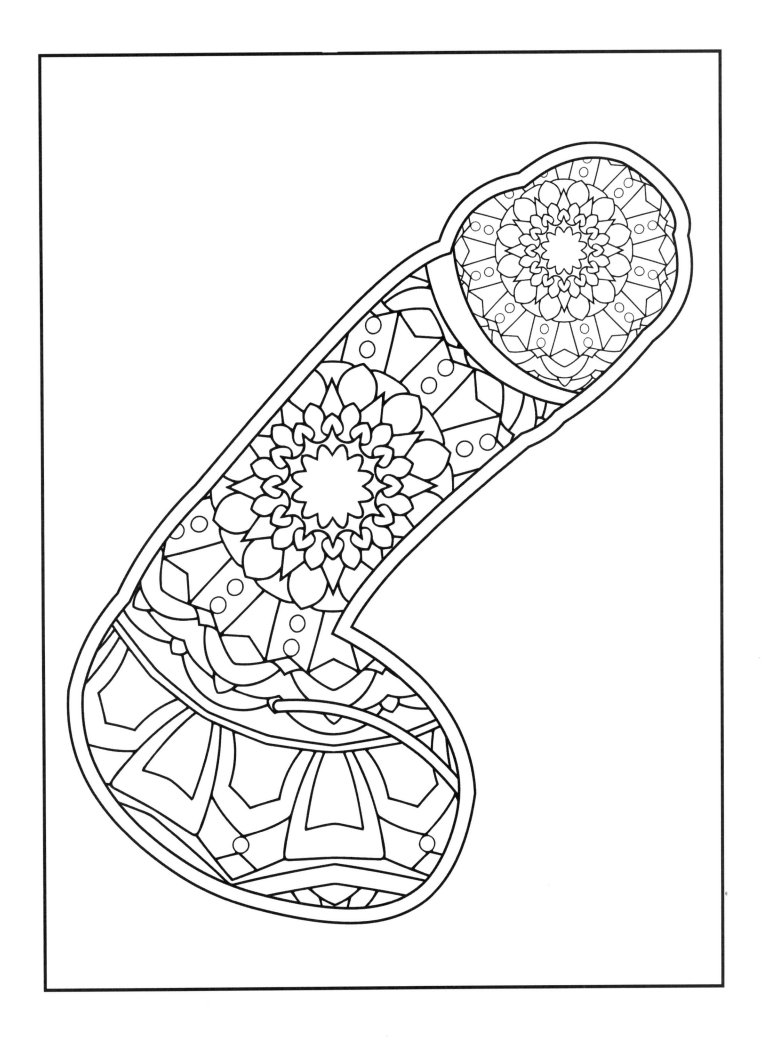

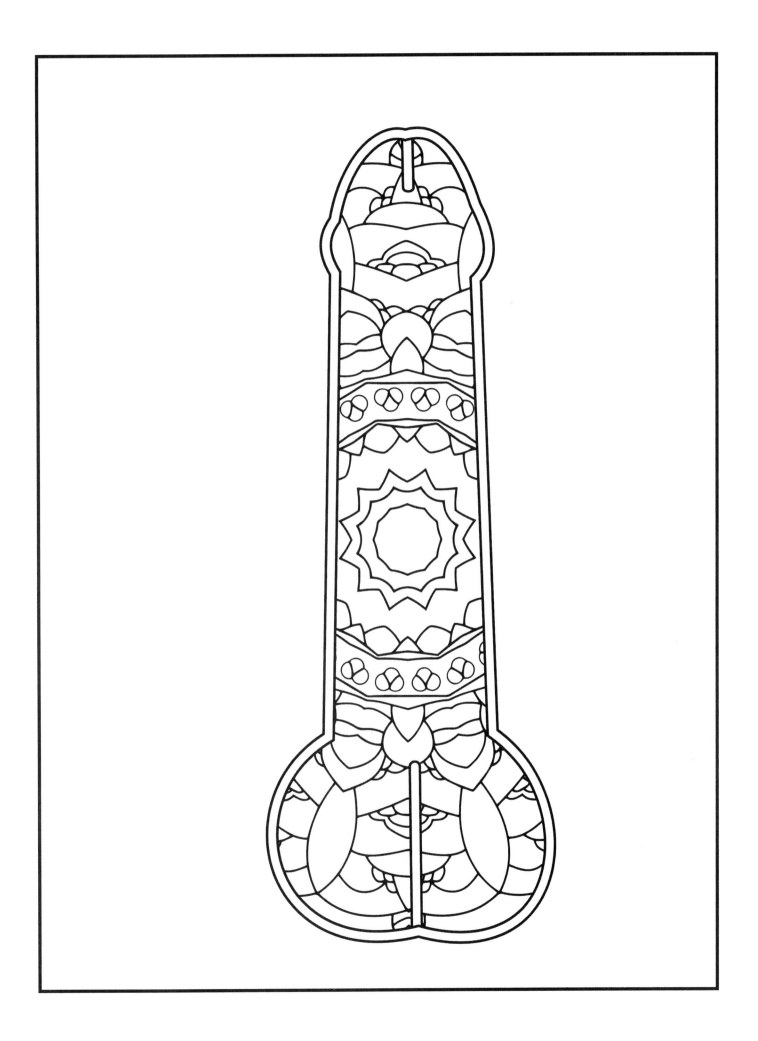

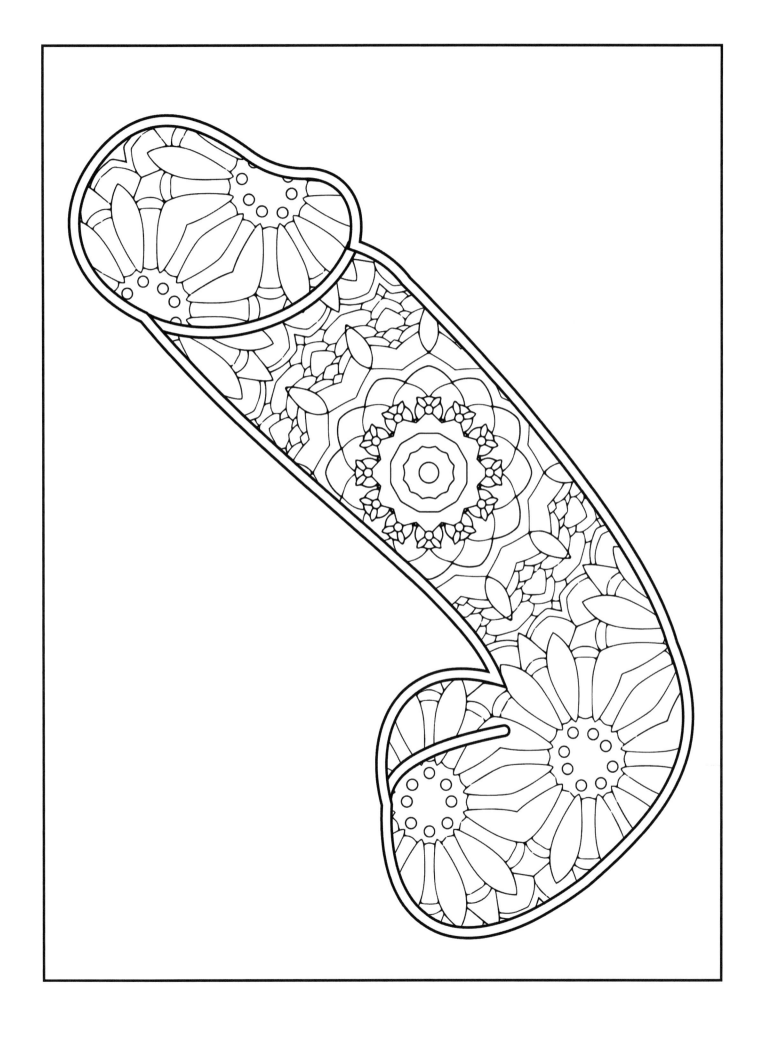

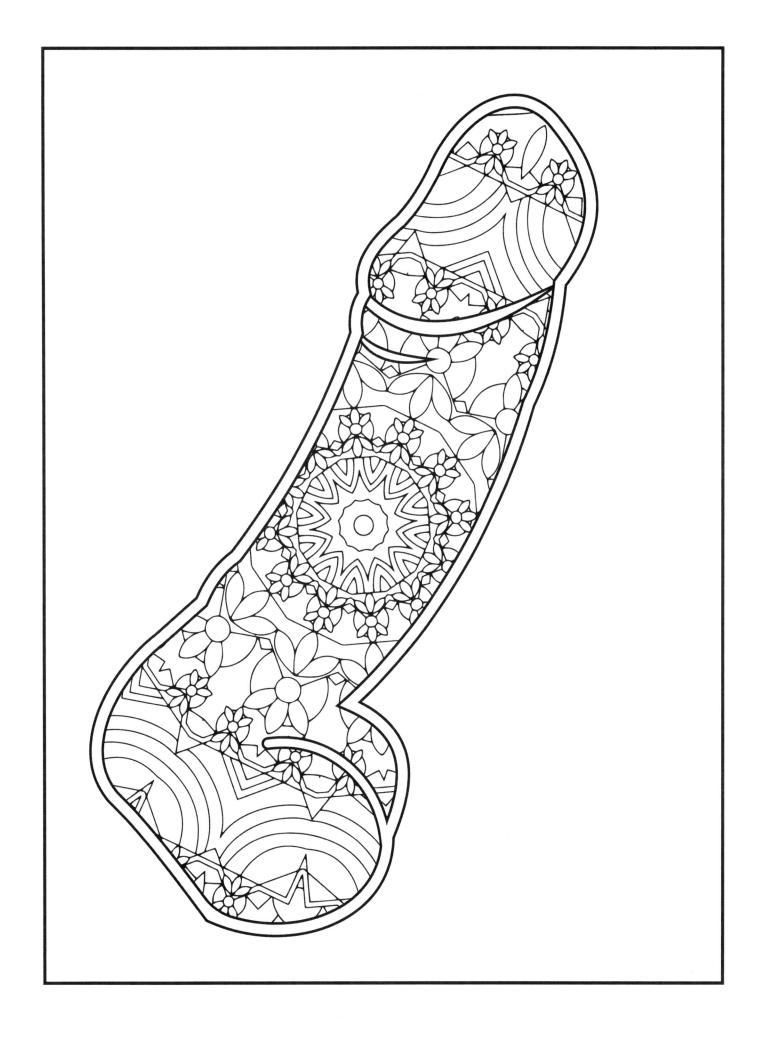

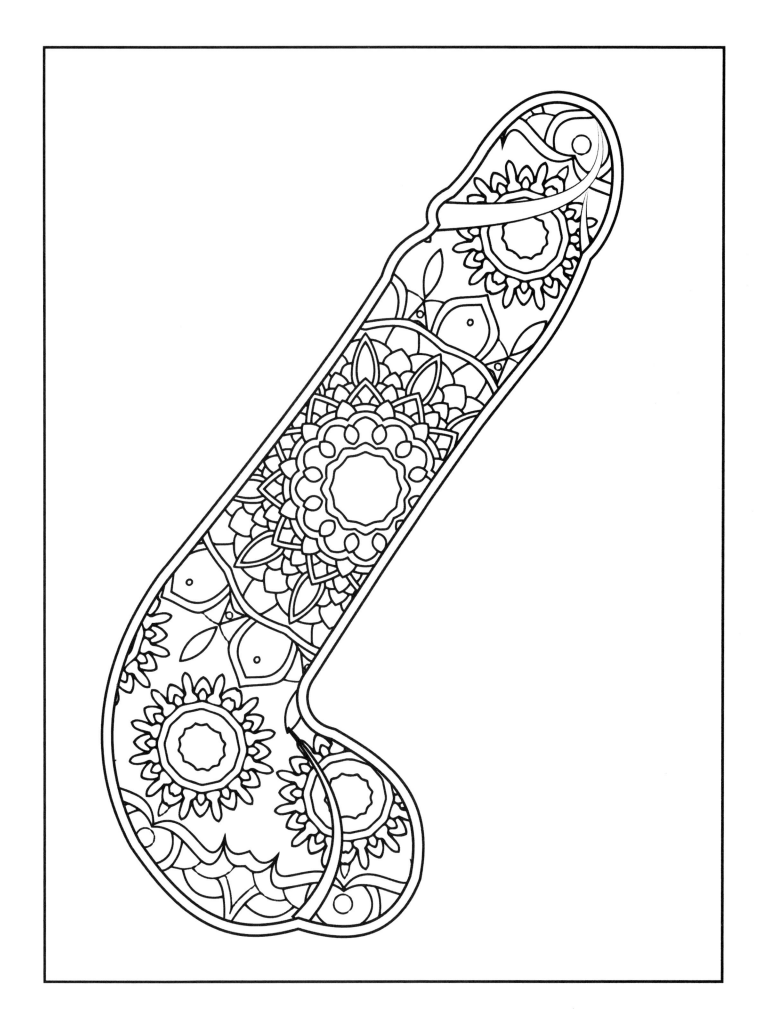

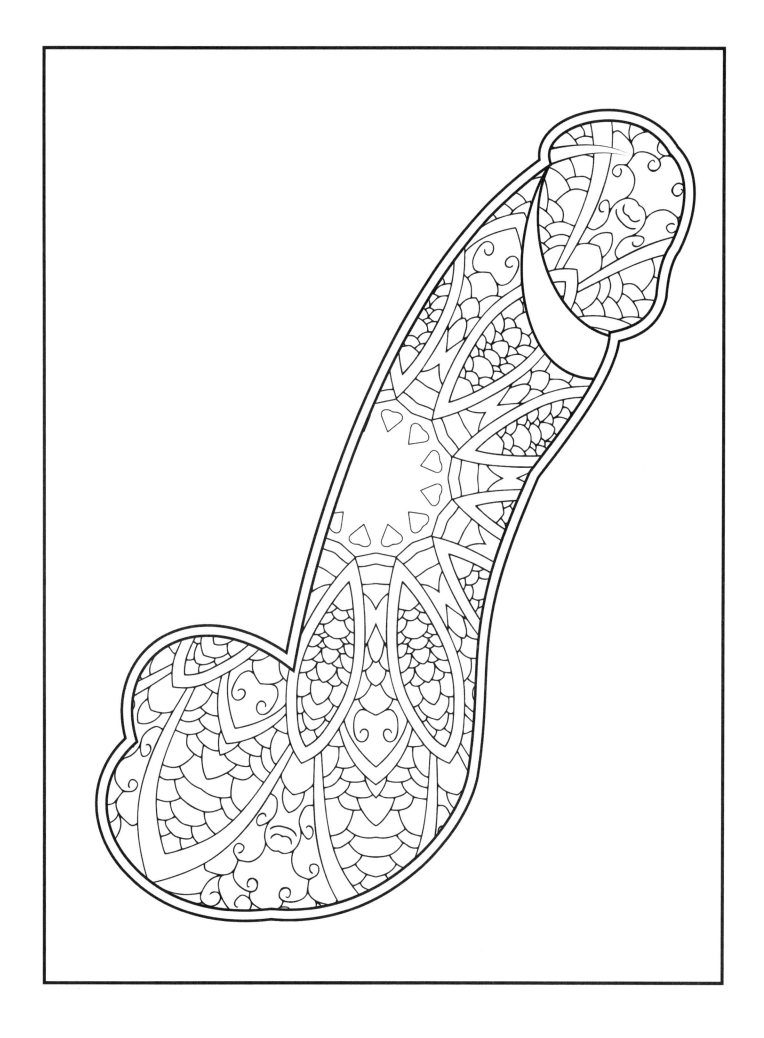

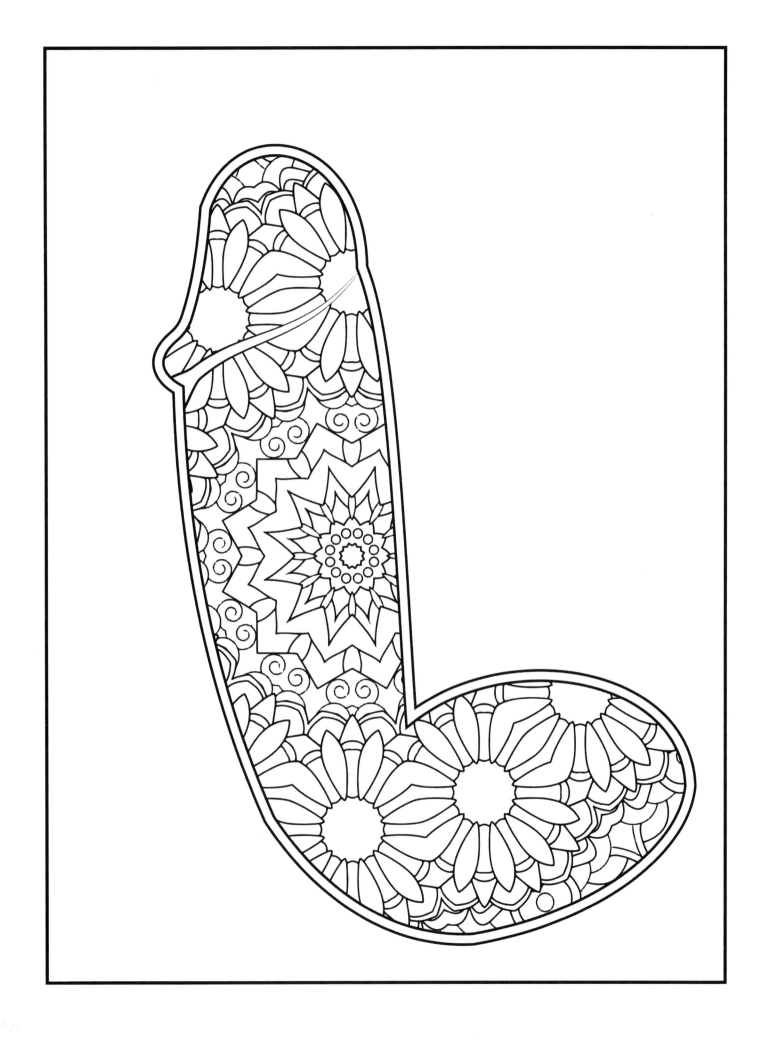

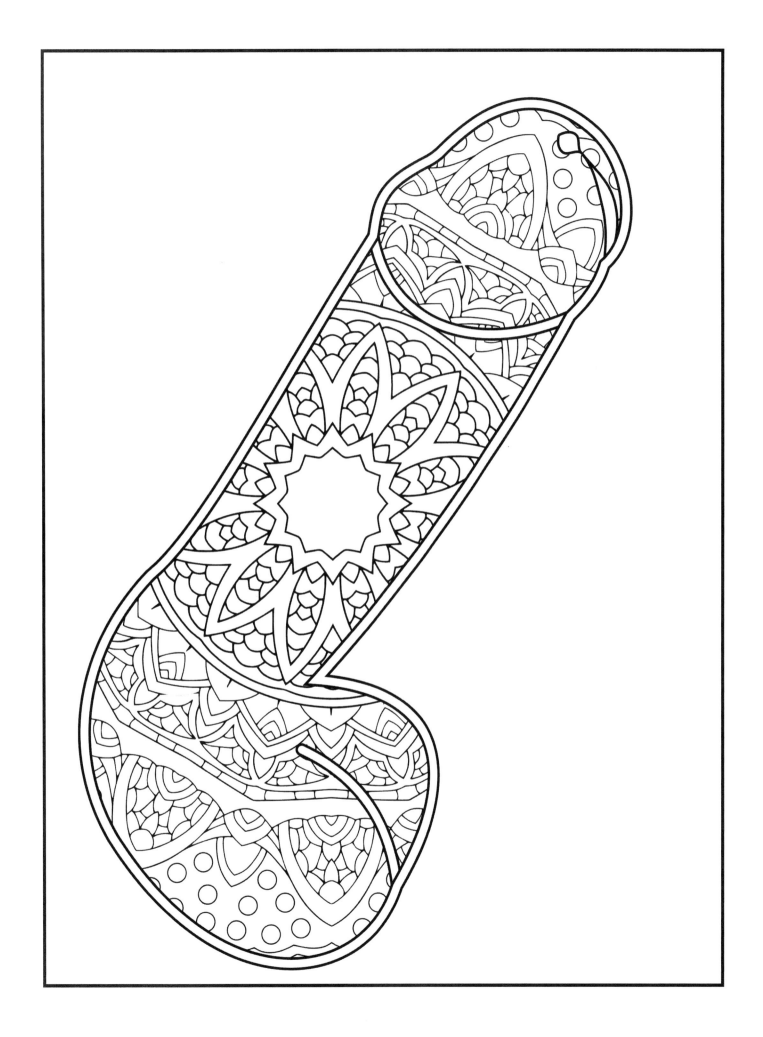

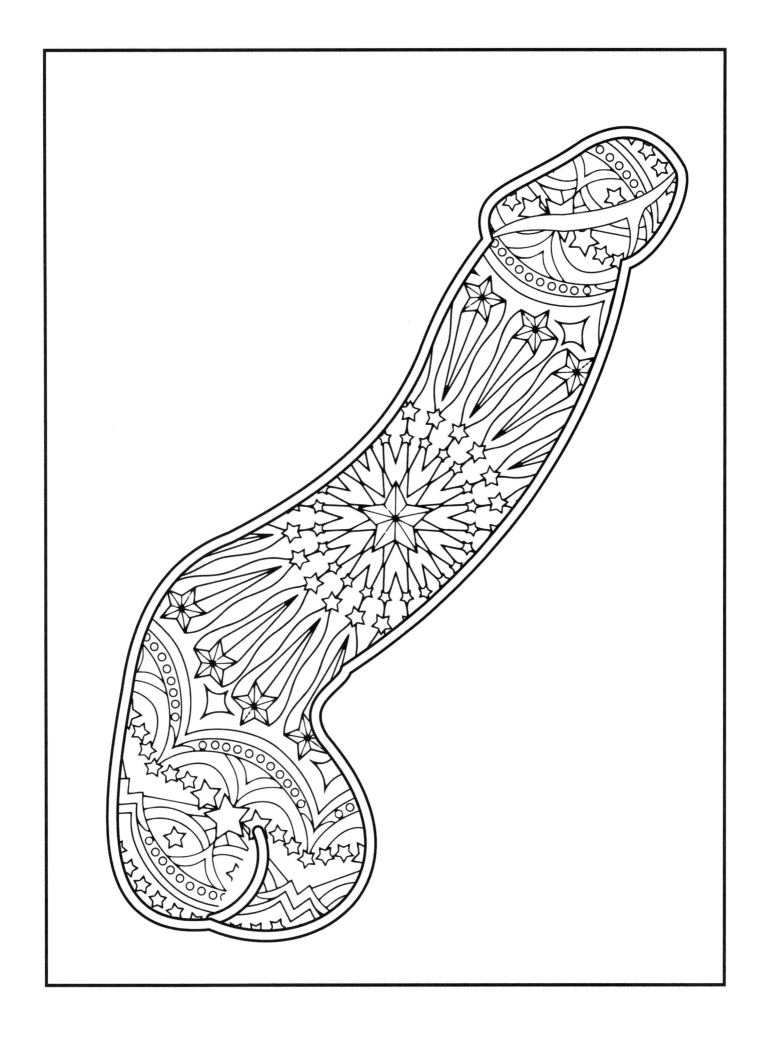

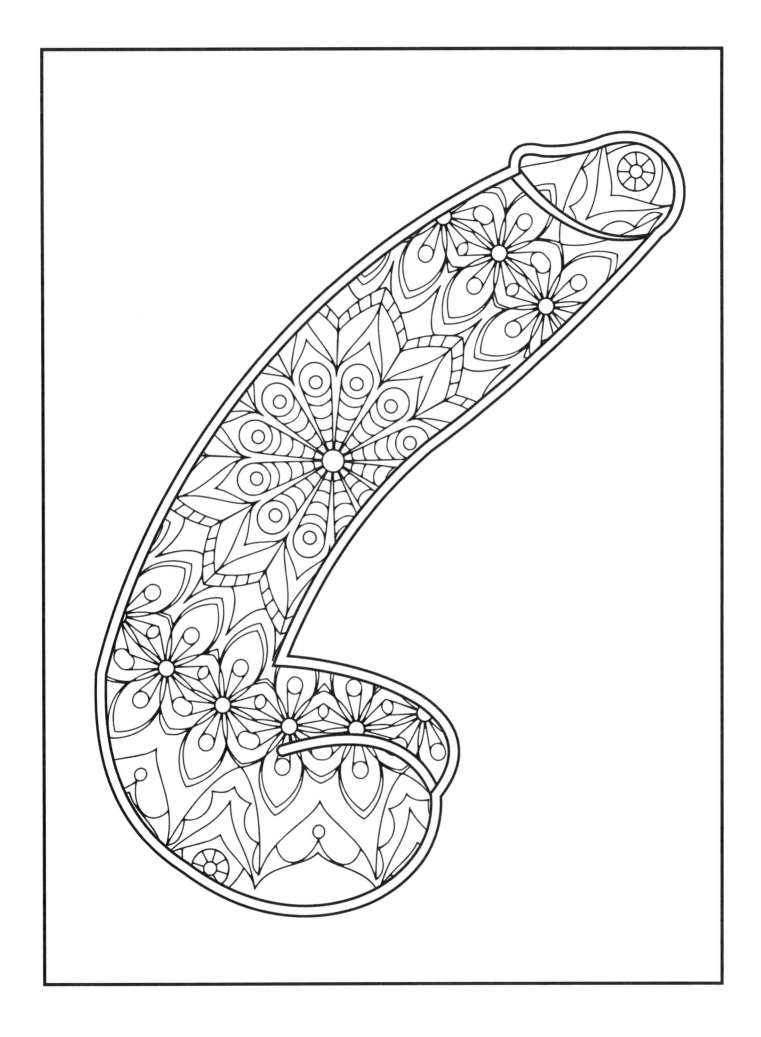

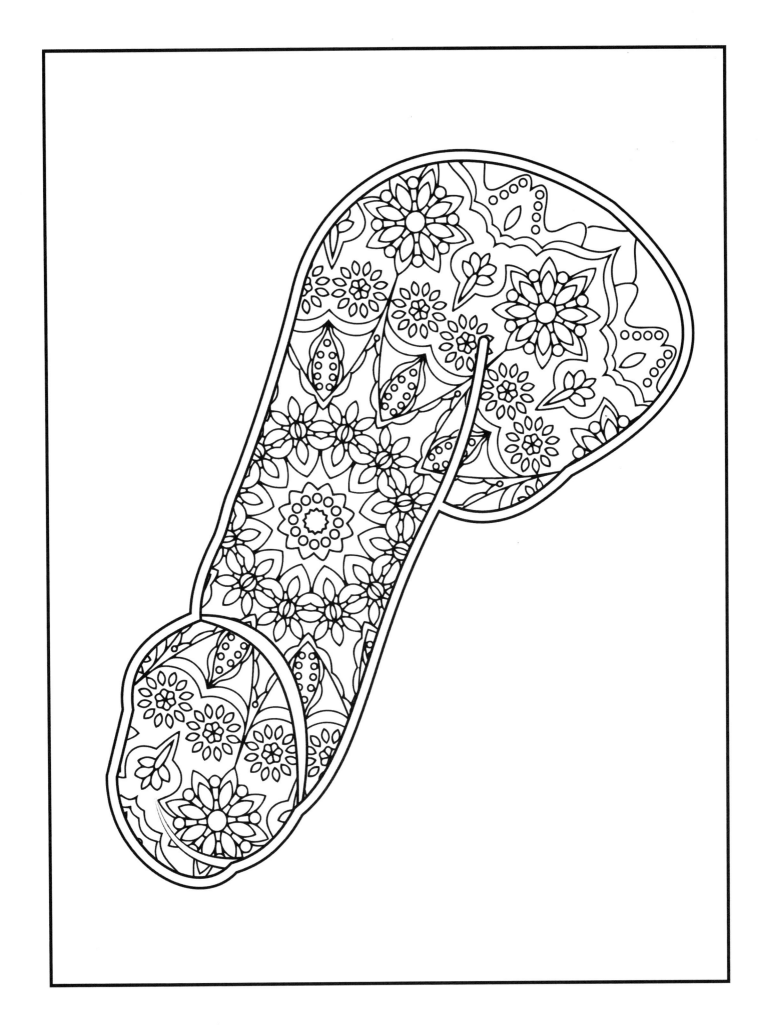

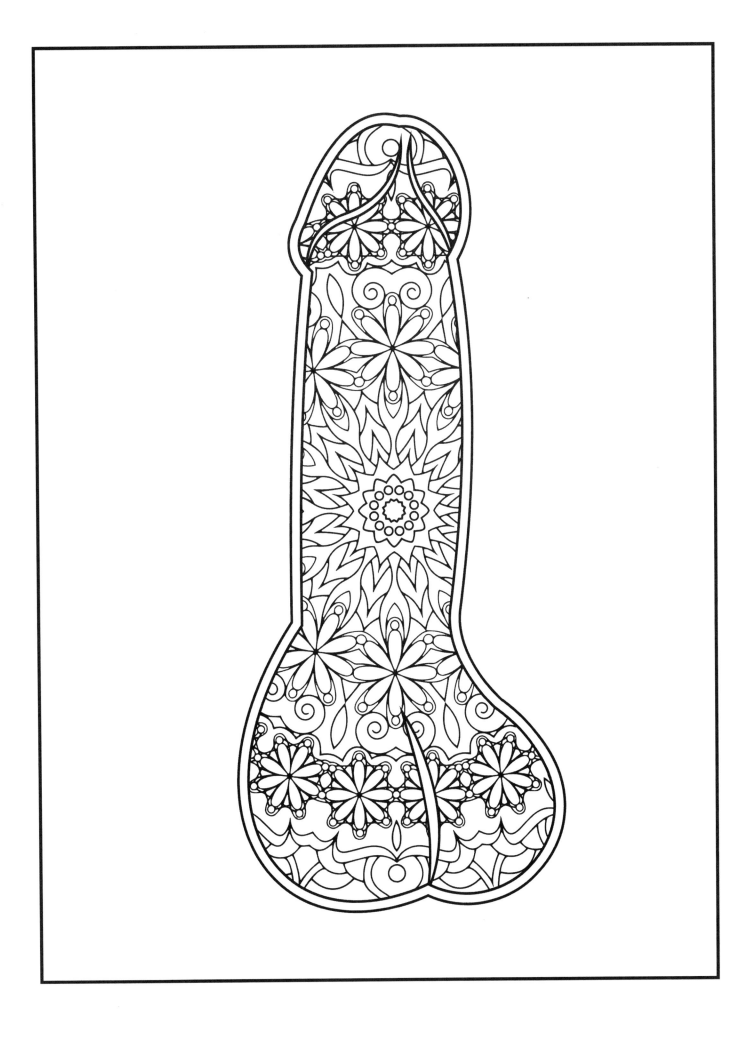

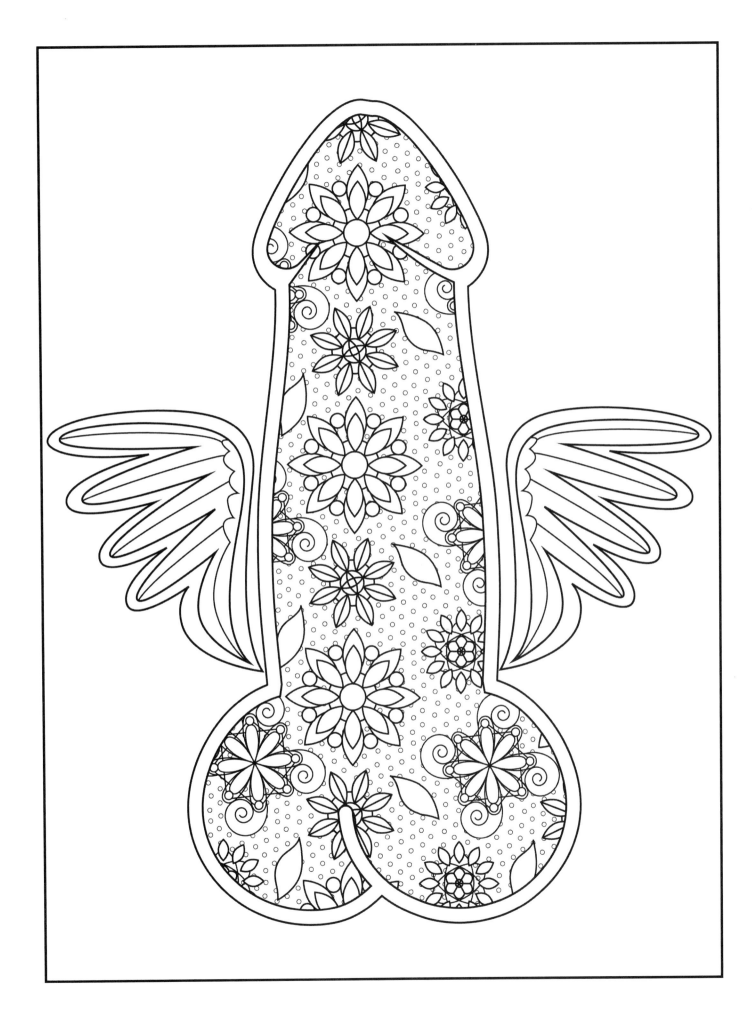

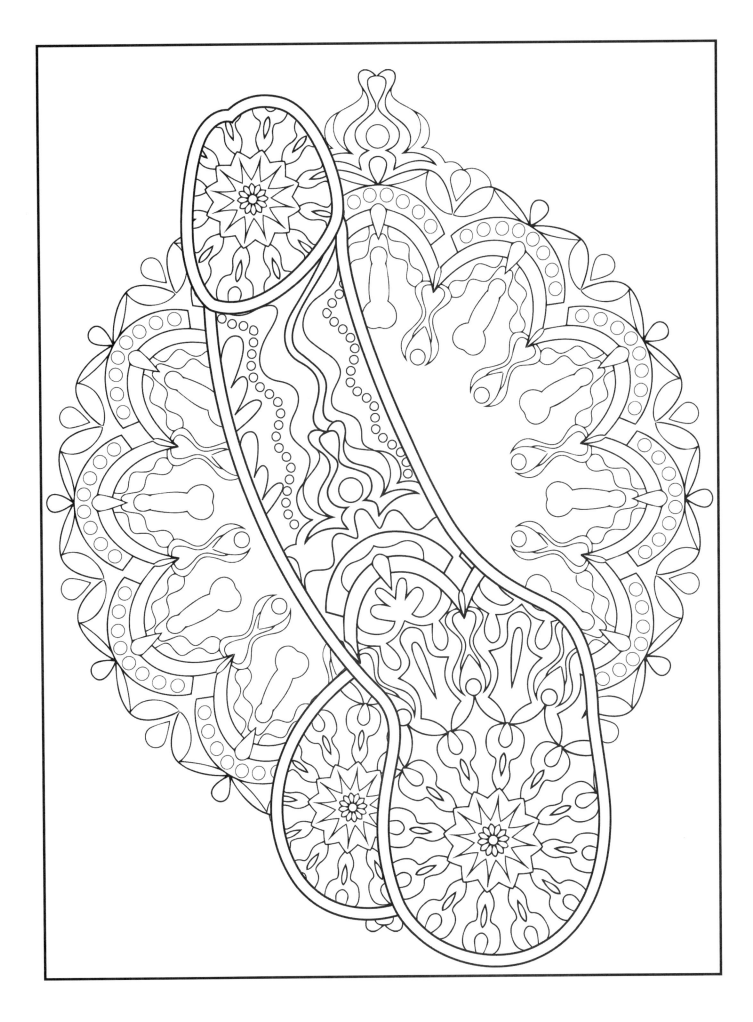

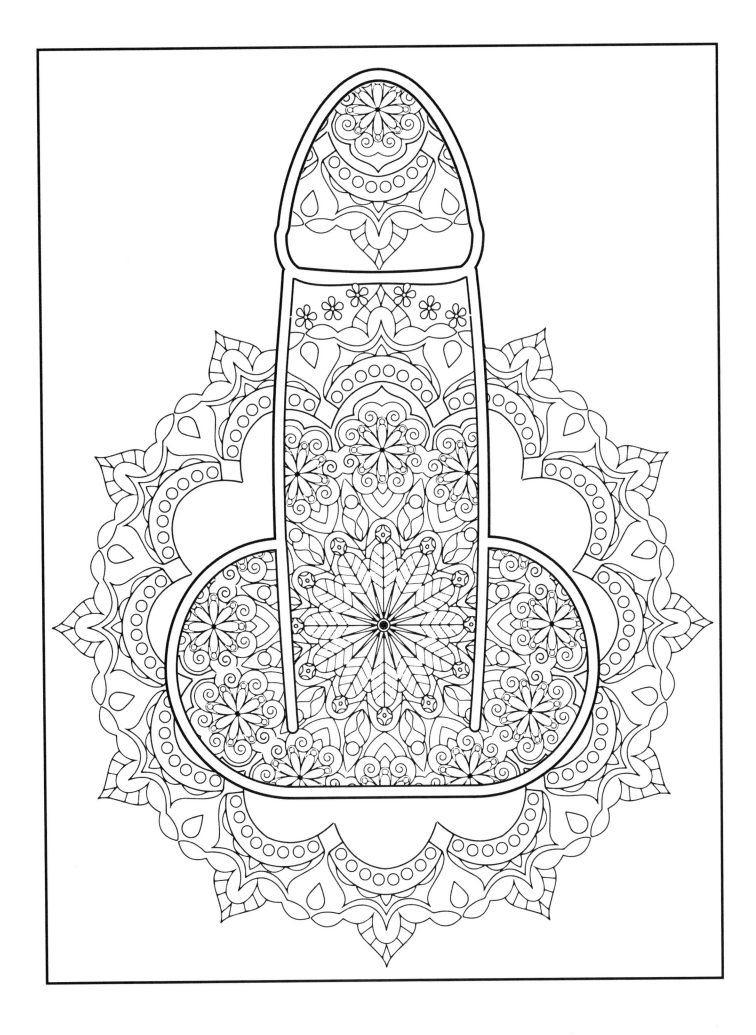

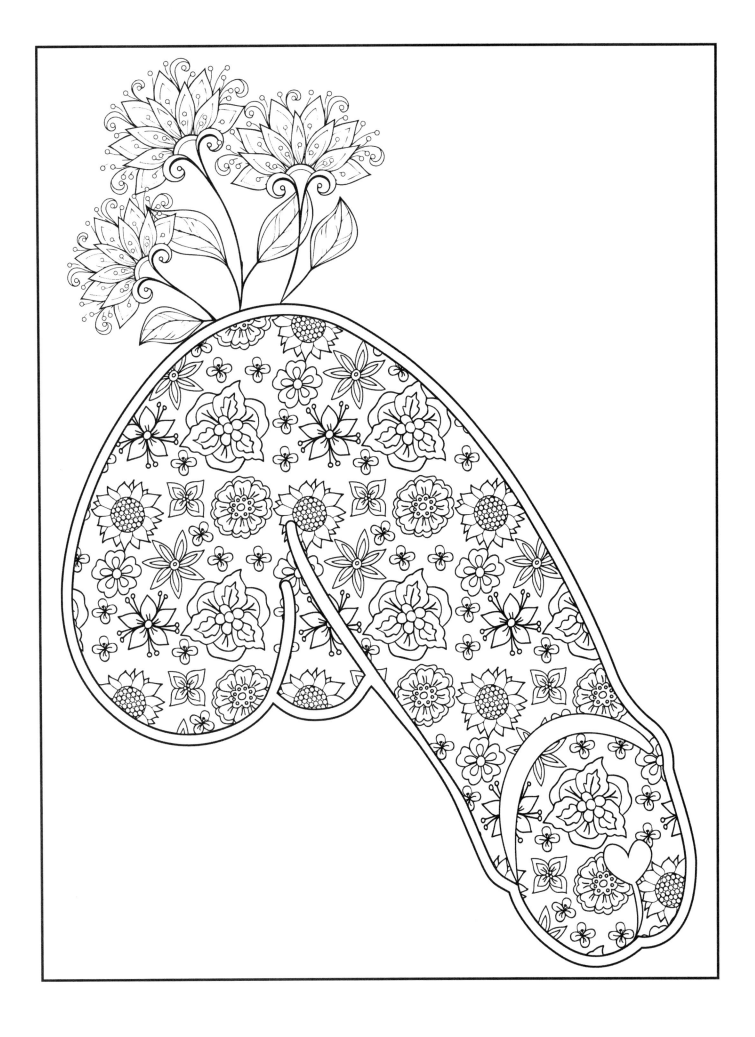

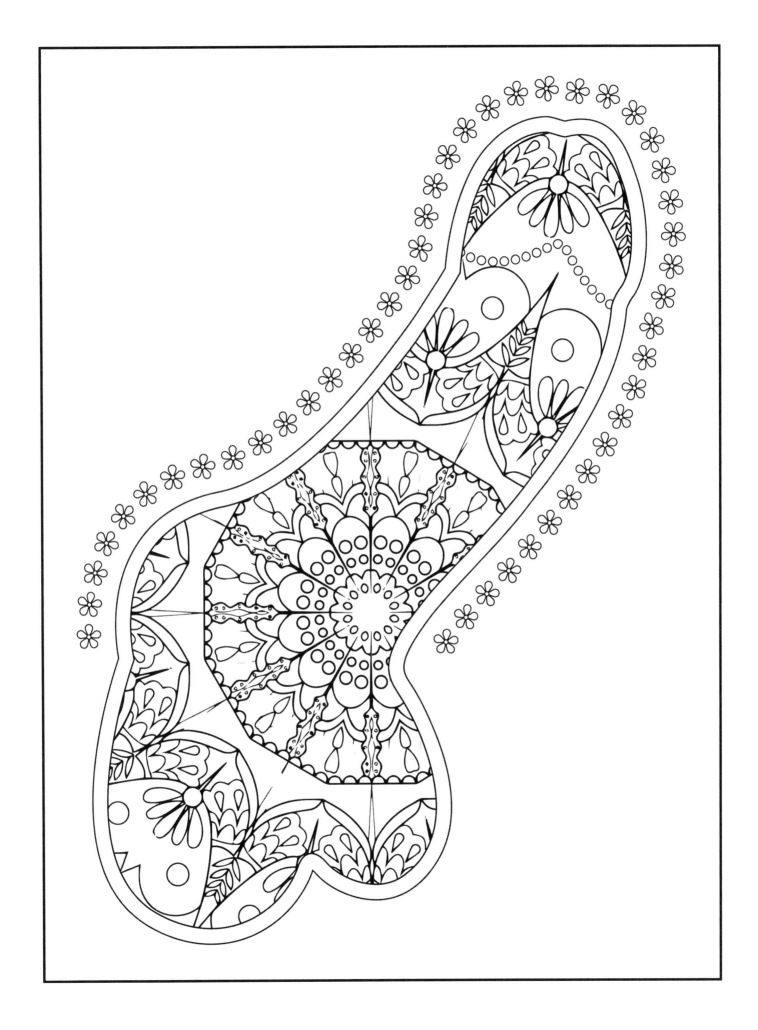

Thank you so much for purchasing this book If you enjoyed it, then please leave an Amazon review. Reviews are the lifeblood of our publishing career. Leaving a positive review would mean the world to us. Cheers!

-Rocco Vidal-

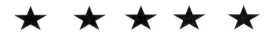